MY REPORT

◀◀◀ **OF** ▶▶▶

FINDINGS

MORE OBSERVATIONS OF A CHIROPRACTIC ADVOCATE

WILLIAM D. ESTEB

Published by Orion Associates, Inc.

Also by William D. Esteb

A Patient's Point of View,
Observations of a Chiropractic Advocate

Beyond Results,
Still More Observations of a Chiropractic Advocate

Making Change,
Even Still More Observations of a Chiropractic Advocate

Published by
Orion Associates, Inc.

Distributed by
Back Talk Systems, Inc.
2845 Ore Mill Drive, Suite 4
Colorado Springs, CO 80904-3161
(719) 633-1105 (800) 937-3113

Cover designed by Buffalo Brothers, Inc.
Manufactured in the United States of America

Esteb, William D., 1952 -

My Report of Findings
More Observations of a Chiropractic Advocate
ISBN 0-9631711-1-9

In memory of Elizabeth Allison Esteb.

CONTENTS

FOREWORD

William Esteb is well acquainted with the various aspects of chiropractic and has written an objective commentary of the profession. For someone who has never enrolled in a chiropractic college, he has extraordinary insight. His practical suggestions have been used in successful offices around the country. This book is not just a commentary dealing with day-to-day practice management, but a manual of essential principles that will prepare chiropractic for the 21st century.

Mr. Esteb is an exceptional and prolific writer and lecturer who has dedicated himself to help elevate the standards of our profession. Chiropractic philosophy will always be the cornerstone of our profession and much of what he ascribes to is based on our cause and effect principle. Raising our personal and professional standards of practice is what *My Report of Findings* is all about.

What follows is a radical departure from the beaten paths which govern the opinions of management consultants currently in vogue. Though at first glance the concepts he advocates may seem unorthodox, his explanations throughout the book are captivating. His ideas are discussed at length and examples are used to illustrate how the intelligent and adaptive practice must prepare to meet the needs of the consumers of the next century. It is essential reading for chiropractors committed to professional excellence and those determined to remain deeply rooted subsequent to any national health care tidal wave. It will make any chiropractor passionately committed to a constant improvement of personal and professional standards.

Bernard Furshpan, D.C.
Bay Shore, New York

1

INTRODUCTION

I consider Bill Esteb the chiropractic Will Rogers of the nineties. His writings reflect the wisdom, wit, and humor that can assist our profession into the next decade.

Times are quickly changing the society we live in and the health care system we work in. In adapting to these changes, the Doctor of Chiropractic has two choices: continue down the dinosaur model of sick patient care or lead the health care sciences into the wellness arena. Bill is prejudiced to the latter and makes a strong case for not only why a wellness practice is necessary, but how to have one.

Each of us is on a journey. Someday we will look back and reflect on the quality of our lives in chiropractic. The quality of our lives and the fulfillment we enjoy is dependent upon the countless decisions we make everyday. If you're looking for a dose of reality combined with an ample amount of encouragement to make better decisions, you won't be disappointed.

You will not find the quick fix that we sometimes think will answer all our problems. Rather you'll be guided through the obstacle course of personal change that will serve as a catalyst to lead you towards the professional success that we all seek.

Claudia Anrig Howe, D.C.
Fresno, California

PREFACE

Even as I was proofing the galleys of my first book, *A Patient's Point of View*, I was continuing to write additional chapter-length magazine articles. As before, the purpose was to think out loud and organize my thoughts. Because each chapter was written as a stand-alone magazine article, certain ideas and subjects are repeated throughout this book as related topics are examined. This is the natural result of exploring a three-dimensional matrix like chiropractic practice in a linear, beginning-middle-and-end format of a book.

Because I am not a Doctor of Chiropractic, my observations here are still from a patient's point of view. If they are helpful, then a great deal of the credit is due to the countless doctors who have invited me to their offices for consultations, and the doctors and their staff who have participated at Permanent New Patient Solution seminars.

Additionally, thank you Dr. Will Tickel for being a sounding board and so generous with your time. Thank you Dr. Claudia Anrig Howe, for your unwavering energy and contagious excitement. Thank you Dr. Bernard Furshpan, for giving form to a big vision for chiropractic. And especially thank you to my partner, Dr. Robert Jackson. Your wisdom and fellowship continue to make a priceless contribution to my life.

Thank you to the Back Talk Systems team, Debbie Richardson, Dusty Sorrentino, Judy Dick, and Megan Kottwitz for making it fun to be in the office and giving me peace of mind when I'm on the road.

Thank you Andrea Ramsauer, for more than 20 years of friendship and offering your considerable editing skills and encouragement in the preparation of this manuscript.

Most of all thank you Marilyn. You honor my dedication to chiropractic and continue to be my worst critic—but my very best friend, wife, and sounding board.

On the following pages I hope I communicate my concern that time is running out to unite, clean house, and prepare for tremendous change in the chiropractic profession. The sense of urgency I feel is real, and so too, I hope, are the suggestions I offer here.

William D. Esteb
Colorado Springs, CO

FIVE ARGUMENTS FOR THE REJECTION OF CHIROPRACTIC

With the recent flurry of media attention chiropractic is receiving, you'd think there would be a line out in front of most chiropractors' offices. But in fact, many offices report their new patient statistics are down. How come?

Those who claim that the television reports and magazine articles have not been positive enough, don't understand how the media works. Actually, to the average viewer or reader, the message has been relatively even handed. Sure, chiropractors hate being relegated to the narrow field of neuromuscular-skeletal specialists, but that is the entry point for today's health care consumer. In another generation, if we play our cards right, that may change. Think of the neuromuscular-skeletal arena as the camel in the old Arabic parable that states, "once the camel's nose is under the tent flap, you can't keep the camel out."

Approaching the general public with the message of the innate healing capacity of each individual and the often wayward character of the educated mind, is not going to win chiropractic a lot of friends. Take the inroads where you can find them! Find a tent flap and push!

Yet even with the welcomed publicity, chiropractic has a long row to hoe to gain the acceptance and utilization most chiropractic doctors dream of. While I'm hopeful, real breakthroughs are unlikely for many years ahead. I hope history proves me wrong, however here are five reasons I'd cite for my lack of optimism:

1. Chiropractic is too low tech. Chiropractic doesn't have the buttons, dials, and digital readouts our culture has become so enamored with. The religion of Scientism that dominates our world today (if you can't touch it, taste it, see it, measure it, etc., it doesn't exist) works against the concept that we are each responsible for our own healing. What do you mean doctors and drugs don't heal the body? The prevailing mechanistic world view makes embracing the holistic chiropractic approach seem primitive and cultish.

Interestingly, at the higher levels of physics where the laws of quantum mechanics are being explored, there is a new respect for the mind/body connection; even the power of thought. Researchers are finding relationships between how they "think" a high energy particle beam experiment will turn out is affecting the results of their experiment. Watch out for what you wish—you may just get it! Until these and other similar observations become mainstream, chiropractic cannot expect to be embraced by the logical, rational, mechanistic keepers of public opinion.

Action steps: Until the world is ready to mend the dichotomy between brain and body, consider collecting a brief synopsis of various research projects. Get a copy of the New Zealand report and highlight important passages for your patients. Subscribe to David Chapman Smith's reports on legal and scientific issues. Have key paragraphs enlarged and posted on a bulletin board reserved for scientific topics. Invest in more technology. Digitized X-rays, EMG, and other forms of technology are often perceived by patients as evidence of "accuracy" and make recommendations more believable. The key is to help your current patients understand the "scientific" nature of chiropractic so they can more successfully combat the attitudes of their friends and families outside your office. Attitude adjustment by communication warfare!

2. Chiropractic lacks instant gratification. Madison Avenue recognizes that when we get a headache, we want "fast, fast relief." The latest products and services advertise the characteristics of "instant", "quick dissolving formula", "microwaveable", and "non-stop service". Time is of the essence. If it isn't fast it must be old. Apparently fast is perceived as stronger, newer, and better.

When chiropractors warn their patients that their problems may actually get worse before they get better, it flies in the face of this prevailing sensitivity to time. When chiropractors explain that it takes time to heal the body, in fact, when certain chronic conditions in adults may require a lifetime of maintenance care to prevent a relapse, it runs counter to a patient's desire for instant gratification.

Action steps: Avoid long waits in your office by more efficient procedures, or at least at a minimum, keep the line moving, even if it's just to another part of your office. Stress patient education. Use a series of progressive examinations to help patients see small increments of progress during the healing process. Ask them what they can do or have been doing, that they hadn't been able to do, before beginning chiropractic care. Ask patients how long they think it takes to heal a broken bone or heal damaged muscle tissue. Remind patients that the long-term aspect of chiropractic care is not the fault of chiropractic, it is the result of the "time clocks" of their own bodies. Place a calendar in your report of findings room for a year or two in the future. "You're probably wondering why I have next year's calendar hanging in my office. It's because many of the patients I'm seeing this year won't start enjoying the real benefits of regular chiropractic until then. The reason for that is because..."

3. Chiropractic is difficult to explain. This may be more problematical than the other reasons because it is dependent upon each practitioner to accomplish. Even offices that smugly report that they use patient education videos, new patient orientation lectures, and a bulging pamphlet rack lack effective patient education. Of course, the litmus test is to ask your patients, "How do you describe what goes on in our office to others?" The answers you hear, even from your best patients, may depress you if you're brave enough to ask. If your best patients can't adequately describe chiropractic, get busy! Since drug companies *won't,* and national chiropractic associations *aren't* providing leadership in this area, it's the responsibility of every doctor.

And it's not just because most patients find it difficult to put the terms "adjustment" and "subluxation" into street language an eighth grader can understand (you try it!). If you were to ask someone on the street what's more important; the heart or the nervous system, nine times out of ten they'll say heart! Check out a typical hospital. Do you think neurologists or brain surgeons rule the roost? No. It's the cardiac boys! The heart specialists are always getting the latest high-tech equipment. Open heart surgery is a real money-maker for most hospitals.

The problem isn't just priorities. It's communications. When patients go to the dentist they can easily describe to others what happened. When patients show up at the hospital for outpatient surgery, they can return home and show others their stitches and explain what happened and why.

Not so with chiropractic. Poor posture, except the most obvious, is rarely noticed by the general public. Poor spinal biomechanics are hidden from view, unlike poor dental health. When orthodontic appliances are purchased, we get to display our financial ability to others—orthodontic braces for adults are the new status symbol. Not so with chiropractic. Your patients are walking the streets and no one can tell they've been to your office.

Action steps: Obviously patient education is the key. Rather than a wordy, oral report of findings, start using more pictures. Bring artifacts into your office so patients can see the barnacles on a rock and rusty antique hinge (subluxation degeneration). Put a dimmer switch in the room where you give your report of findings. Make more of your patient education effort experiential. Patients aren't reading your wordy brochures. They're not remembering the eloquent words spoken during your report.

4. Chiropractic has a poor public image. Although many chiropractors have lost touch with some of the prevailing attitudes about chiropractic, the profession and it's practitioners still have a tarnished public image. Being perceived as an "alternative" non-mainstream healing "art", with its bearded, charismatic, and uneducated-white-leather-plaid-polyester "doctors" is a severe handicap. Rarely does today's chiropractic student choose chiropractic because they couldn't get into medical school, yet the stigma of being less than a "real" doctor remains. The image of chiropractic is a serious fault at a time when the "quality" of a product or service is often more important than the price. Many of us willingly pay extra for the quality of brand name products.

This creates a damaging form of peer pressure in which many of your patients, even those who get great results from your care, are unwilling to divulge to others that they consulted your office. These are the same people who at home, pour less expensive scotch into their expensive brand name bottles and announce to the world on their license plate that "my other car is a BMW". Image and style has become substance. Being associated with an "alternative healing art" is a reflection of poor judgment or the lack of financial resources. The "chiropractic underground" continues to thrive.

Those who argue that this attitude is changing are right. Disappointment with the medical model and an avoidance of drugs and surgery are helping attract patients to chiropractic. Yet for many, they aren't necessarily "voting" for chiropractic, they are simply voting against medicine.

Action steps: Explain to your patients the decision-making process you went through when deciding to become a chiropractic doctor. Then, set a good example in everything you say and do. Current patients and potential patients in your community are watching your actions, studying your habits, analyzing the decisions you make, and judging your appearance. Avoid short-term promotional strategies that sabotage your professional stature. Since changing these perceptions of chiropractic should start in your office, ask each patient "what do you think the general public's biggest misconception about chiropractic is?" Since they won't be able to consult the latest Gallup poll, their answer is most likely going to be what their own biggest misconception is. "And how do you explain to others that that misconception is inaccurate?" you ask as a follow up question. Make sure your own patients can properly defend the misconceptions they encounter. Make your patients more resourceful should the opportunity to mention, explain, or defend chiropractic presents itself in their sphere of influence.

5. Chiropractic is expensive. While it's true countless research studies indicate that chiropractic care is more effective and less expensive than other forms of care for similar conditions, this information is lost on the general public. Influenced heavily by the insurance industry, most chiropractic doctors have fashioned a fee policy in the upper limits of what this sickness care industry will pay. Suddenly we have adjustments costing as much as $25, $35, $45, or higher, depending upon where you practice. If only one or two adjustments were needed, this probably would fly. But when prospective patients learn that months or years of repeated visits are needed (once you start going you have to go for the rest of your life), the perceived cost of care becomes a major limiting factor.

Today, as the insurance industry crumbles, this is an even more important concern. If after every $45 adjustment the patient saw radical physiological changes in their body; a "tingling" that lasted for days or at least hours afterwards—no problem. But after the first few visits, the effect is more subtle. Sure, there are those who will continue their care for the rest of their lives because "it feels good", but this is a small part of your practice.

Setting a fee structure that is responsive to the budget constraints of today's economic realities is a major challenge for most doctors. This is especially difficult for doctors and staff, who get their care without impact to their monthly budget, to understand.

Action steps: Become more resourceful in the presentation of your financial policies by having more organized options to offer. Perhaps develop a case management fee (as long as you don't imply cure) and a wellness fee arrangement (unlimited wellness care for a fixed monthly fee). Brainstorm what you'd change, if tomorrow all insurance coverage for chiropractic was rescinded in your state. Start making changes now!

You can't afford the luxury to take a single new patient for granted. Patients bold enough to try chiropractic are often doing so based on the encouragement of a trusted friend or the patient education efforts of someone you haven't even met. They're desperate. They're afraid. And they're bucking the establishment. Many are coming to your office with misgivings and questioning their own judgment. If you have relatives who still don't accept, understand, or respect what you do, then you understand how many of these new patients are suffering. ■

A DOCTOR'S REPUTATION

How is it that medical doctors, with their crude attempts at finding a chemical solution to every disease of the body (or removing the offending part) became accepted? And how is it that the chiropractic doctor, with their location and correction of the cause of disease has remained largely unrespected and ignored? How did this happen and how can this injustice be reversed?

Like lawyers of the 17th and 18th century, doctors were among the most educated and respected in their communities. These were individuals who had a larger world view than the farmers and simple shop keepers of the time. This was an era in which a large portion of the world was tied to the land, either as farmers or herders of domesticated animals. Only the children of large land owners and the very rich could afford a college education. Becoming a professional and giving back to the community in the form of legal help or medical aid, was seen as the duty of many in this elite class. In fact, many spurned payment of any kind for their services.

Simultaneous with the emergence of the legal and medical professional, there were profound changes in the religious and intellectual climate in Western Europe. Dissection of the human body was prevented by the powerful Catholic church until 1733, preventing even the most rudimentary understanding of bodily function! This was the time of Galileo, Newton, Copernicus, and others who, with the telescope, mathematics, and new intellectual freedoms, produced a mechanistic view of the world that remained in place well into the recent past, with the acceptance of an Einsteinian view of the world. Even the theories of Darwin contain somewhat of a mechanistic, form follows function ideology. As the Industrial Age dawned in the early 1800s, the physiology of the human body became heavily influenced by this prevailing world view. Like interchangeable gun parts that allowed mass production methods, the body was seen as a complex machine with individual and separate parts. Disease and ill-health was not seen as a whole body phenomenon, but as an isolated part that was broken, wearing out, or somehow out of step with the rest of the body. Medicine was seen as the way to "speed up" organs or systems that were not functioning enough or "slowing down" organs or systems that were functioning too much. Chemistry was seen as the management tool to tend the human machine.

While the Industrial Age did free some from the 18 hour days of back-breaking soil tending, most people became harnessed to factory machines instead. This continued to isolate more and more people from the time and financial resources necessary to attend schools of higher learning and escape the exploitation that a lack of education produced. Besides the lack of understanding the general public (and doctors of the time) had of human physiology, sanitary standards were still woefully absent. Besides providing fertile conditions for TB, and other infectious diseases, it became a compelling environment for the germ theory to emerge. Suddenly it became accepted that germs were the cause of disease. This theory so easily explained the prevailing, cause-effect, mechanistic view of the world that was obvious to the five senses. Sick people had obvious symptoms and "germs" were present.

Vaccinations seemed the perfect solution to this menace and countless millions had their immune systems modified to combat the threat of invisible viruses. And it seemed to work. No matter that simultaneously sanitary conditions improved and better personal hygiene became more prevalent, there seemed a statistically measurable reduction in communicable diseases and vaccinations received the credit.

The scientific method, with control groups and placebos gave the culture something to cling to. There became a growing mistrust of the body and its propensity to sin and generate unclean thoughts, and most

14

of the Western world saw a religious revival of huge proportion. It was estimated that in the mid-1800s that as much as 80% of the population were regular church-goers. (Today that figure is closer to half as many.) As ill-health and disease were seen as something caused by outside sources, it became more and more accepted that solutions should come from outside the body too.

As we entered the early 1900s, the curriculum of medical schools, which at the time included less than a year of formal education, became more comprehensive. More schooling was required as more and more combinations and permutations of diseases were discovered, documented, and chemical or surgical interventions (outside forces) were devised to combat them. Ultimately this system produced specialists who limited their careers to understanding narrow aspects of human physiology and pathology.

As the germ theory became more and more entrenched, diagnosing and learning the countless therapies used to combat "the enemy" made medical school increasingly expensive and reserved for the best and the brightest. It became somewhat of a cliché that the highest hope a mother could have for her son, was to become a doctor and join the ranks of the country's most elite and respected professional class. This class distinction, while not as tyrannical as the caste system of India, created a privileged few who were granted access to increasingly powerful drugs and the skills of surgical intervention.

Doctors knowingly or unknowingly exploited this advantage over their patients. With authority they prescribed and directed patient behavior without question (doctor's orders). The general population, with their ignorance of even the most fundamental human physiology were grateful even to see a doctor. The medical doctor's words were taken as gospel, without reservation. Patients willingly waited for hours for a brief encounter with the all knowing doctor who had, at considerable personal sacrifice, performed the required book learning and internship to be granted the responsibility of shepherding a practice of patients through the unseen dangers of a disease-filled world. Nature became the enemy.

With the demands placed upon these few anointed individuals, patient "management" practices were adopted to increase efficiency.

Patients routinely waited in magazine-filled reception rooms. Births were routinely induced to the more convenient schedule of the treating doctor. More and more technology, more and more tests, and more and more invasive procedures were used. Low tech solutions were spurned, and more and more respect (and dependence) was given to technological breakthroughs. Powerful antibiotics, organ transplants, DNA splicing, in utero-micro surgery, test tube babies, and other exotic procedures first made front page news, and then became routine and expected. If problems didn't respond to the high-tech approach, it became the patient's fault or it was all in the patient's head.

And then things started to change. The baby boom generation emerged. In the United States over 76 million strong, they became the most educated group in history. They changed the world in a most profound way. They questioned authority figures in all disciplines. They asked questions. Their favorite? "Why?" They sought second opinions. They became a generation accustomed to medical miracles, chemical birth control, polio vaccinations, antibiotics, and routine medical success stories. This same generation is watching their parents die of cancers, hypertension, heart disease, and countless preventable lifestyle diseases that don't seem to fit the germ theory model.

While there are exceptions, this generation has more of a potential to be available to the chiropractic message than any before it. If chiropractic is going to assume its rightful place in the health care sciences, it must act on the opportunity presented by the emergence of the baby boom generation. How are you making "low-tech" health care approaches (like chiropractic), attractive to this highly-educated generation weaned on a medical model of health? ■

PRIME TIME CHIROPRACTIC

The medical model of health has permeated our culture to such a degree, that most doctors of chiropractic fight an uphill battle to get patients to understand how chiropractic differs from medicine. Some doctors have given up and don't even try anymore. Good communication skills are necessary and it takes time and energy to conduct this effort patient by patient. A new patient orientation lecture and report of findings are likely to be insufficient to do the complete job. An entire lifetime steeped in the medical approach isn't replaced in a couple of chiropractic visits, even with excellent clinical results.

Just inspect *TV Guide* during prime time television for the last 30 years! Look what's inside the hidden recesses of the cerebral cortex of your next 43-year old low back patient. Imagine how strange chiropractic philosophy must appear to patients who have been trained so well by television.

Although a few medical doctor shows appeared in the 1950's, *Ben Casey* started airing in 1961 and in its five year run, set the stage for medical drama. Played by Vince Edwards, his good looks and medical expertise thrilled an entire generation of patients. How many of your patients, who as teenagers, had crushes on this attractive man who seemed to have an answer for everything?

Also airing in 1961 was *Dr. Kildare*, set at Blair General Hospital. Richard Chamberlain played the title role for six years. Again, the casting and story line put medicine into a glamorous light, replacing westerns and providing a new source of heroes for a growing baby boom generation. Difficult health problems, often the result of a lifetime of neglect, were wrapped up neatly with a bow in an hour. No wonder every mother's dream was to have her son grow up to become a doctor. A real doctor.

Happy endings were the trademark of another popular doctor show that premiered in the fall of 1969. Robert Young began starring in the lead role of *Marcus Welby, M.D.* It became one of television's most successful medical dramas, running for seven seasons on ABC. This gentle father figure was so attractive to viewers, and the apparent line between reality and mythology so vague, Young received thousands of letters each month requesting medical advice!

Before *Marcus Welby* left the air, the irreverent *M*A*S*H* began airing. A black comedy based on the movie and successful book, this popular show always featured at least one operating room sequence. With few exceptions, these doctors were able to find the problem, correct it, and send the patient back to the states or back to the front line. While many of the themes in this successfully syndicated program poked fun at the military, the horrors of war, or explored the personality flaws of those under stress, the "doctor in charge" attitude permeated every show. And while it was entertaining to watch the doctors' unusual or humorous antics, somehow the patient pulled through, or there was a warm feeling created by the all knowing doctor righting a wrong or solving a difficult problem.

This same "medical doctor in control" image was exhibited in the *Six Million Dollar Man*, a story about a human with man-made parts. Here, the medical model saw its finest hour, subverting the minds of millions of viewers so that they believed medical intervention not only could repair the body, but also could somehow improve human function! Sound effects and dramatic slow motion sequences emphasized these inhuman qualities. Ultimately every Ken doll needs a Barbie and the *Bionic Woman* joined the medical marvel to solve crime and do things the rest of us couldn't do. Every week the opening sequence of this popular prime time entertainment taught us that medicine could make us more complete.

18

More recently, *St. Elsewhere, Quincy, China Beach, Doogie Houser, M.D.,* and others have used the medical setting to do everything from solving crimes to provide an entertaining vehicle to explore relationships. Add to these, the countless emergency medicine "911" shows and the sappy daytime soap operas, and you have hours of television programming that directly sanction and endorse the medical model of health.

And it's not just the medical setting. Because of the time restraints of television and the desire to leave viewers with every loose end accounted for, even the most tragic health care problems find painless resolution. In 23 minutes plus commercials, everything from cancer to drug addiction has a happy ending. It's clean, controlled, and sterile. Medicine seems to have the answer for any human shortcoming. Apparently health solutions come from the test tube, the hypodermic, good timing, finding a caring doctor, or the surgeon's hands. Not from the patient's own innate healing ability.

That's just the programming. The real soap operas are the ones lasting thirty seconds, promising relief from headaches, backaches, and every other ailment even remotely socially acceptable to discuss in a prime-time setting. The mind-numbing frequency that ads for these analgesics are seen by your patients is enough to give them the conditions they are designed to treat! (Funny, the same chiropractic doctors who complain the loudest about this medical clutter in prime time are often the same ones who allow magazines in their reception room to advertise the very same products!)

So how about a prime time chiropractic television show?

Ignore for a moment the medical advertisers that would prevent a show devoted to chiropractic from ever seeing the light of the phosphorous screen. What would a dramatic one-hour TV show look like that endorsed the chiropractic philosophy?

Fade up on a rain-slicked city street at night. Over dramatic theme music, super title: "Doctor, Doctor" to which is added: "VSC: The Silent Killer." Zoom into chiropractic office late at night. Music continues as we see the doctor working late, dictating a report at his desk. Music fades under as the doctor gets up from his desk and continues his dictation as he walks to the X-ray view box. Lighting from the X-ray view box gives

19

the rugged lines and chiseled features of the doctor's face a wise, but approachable demeanor.

Cut to a family in a station wagon coming home from shopping. Headlights cut into the camera lens and we hear the sounds of laughing children. Cut to a drunk driver weaving down the road in same direction. Cut back and forth between both drivers and the approaching stop sign. Music builds tension as the station wagon pulls up to the stop sign and the mother is unaware of the drunk driver bearing down upon her from the rear. Cut to fast cuts of slow motion footage of the cars colliding as we see the driver and children suffer serious whiplash injuries.

Cut to the busy chiropractic reception room the next morning. The telephone rings and it is answered by the receptionist, "Smith Relief and Wellness Clinic, this is Nancy, may I help you?"

See where this plot line is going? The mother and children survived the automobile accident but are going to need a generous amount of Initial Intensive Care, and the real drama is whether they have uninsured motorist coverage and how large their deductible is! The subplot involves a skeptical husband who was in an accident and the pain went away on its own after a couple of days. No high technology solutions. No untested miracle drugs. Just 20 or 30 visits that last about five minutes and look amazingly the same from visit to visit. Where's the compelling life or death drama? Since chiropractic patients are reminded that they are doing the healing, not the doctor, the team of surgeons struggling to subdue the evil forces of disease are absent.

Maybe a half-hour sitcom would be a better format instead.

Fade up on a busy reception room as the exam doctor pops his head into the doctor's private office as he is completing a narrative. "Hey Bob, Mrs. Johnson's X-rays are in the processor and she's ready in adjusting room two. Oh, by the way, did I tell you the one about the lawyers and the tooth fairy?" Cut to disinterested doctor folding a patient file and getting up to take down a set of X-rays from view box. Cut to wide shot of both doctors as exam doctor continues with his joke. "Well, there are these three guys sitting around a table, an expensive lawyer, an inexpensive lawyer, and the tooth fairy." Cut to doctor's "oh-no-here-we-go-again" reaction shot. Exam doctor continues. "On the table is fifty bucks. Suddenly, the lights go out for just a few seconds. When they come back on, the fifty dollars is missing." The doctor has taken down all the X-rays, put them in the file, and is leaving the room to the front desk. The exam doctor tags along behind the doctor and continues with his joke. "The question is, who took the fifty bucks?" "I don't know, who took the 50 dollars," says the doctor disinterestedly as he turns to the receptionist, "How many do we have scheduled this afternoon, Nancy?" The exam doctor explodes with the punch line, "The expensive lawyer of course, because we all know there's no such thing as the tooth fairy or an inexpensive lawyer." Laugh track is heard as we see several patients react as they look up from reading their magazines. Theme music up as show title supers over live action.

Or how about a chiropractic based game show?

Naw.

Somehow the intuitive, non-linear aspects of chiropractic don't translate easily into the format we're accustomed to seeing on television. Showing a cervical chiropractic adjustment on television is more difficult to understand and appreciate than drugs, surgery, or even physical therapy. In fact, demonstrating an adjustment is often counter-productive because it looks more traumatic to the viewer than it is to the patient. The 10% or so of the population familiar with the procedure would understand, yet that's hardly enough viewership to build a television audience.

Instead, we have amateurs creating chiropractic television commercials. These 30-second attempts at new patient solicitation help form the image of chiropractic for millions of people. Juxtaposed among the high-budget McDonald's commercials and other national spots, chiropractic advertising often projects a sleazy, unprofessional image. And it's too bad. Because it won't be until chiropractic can effectively penetrate and exploit the media of television or film that it will be able to assume its rightful place in the healing arts. ■

HONORING THE PATIENT

Actor William Hurt's character, the hot shot surgeon in the movie *The Doctor*, found the tables turned when he became a cancer patient. He discovered the insensitivity displayed by the reams of paperwork, unexplained waiting, and uncommunicative doctors and staff to be dehumanizing. Even in the busiest offices, chiropractic rarely approaches even the most modest examples portrayed in the movie. Yet, since many patients have considered chiropractic as a last resort and have heard countless horror stories about the profession, they may feel just as alone and apprehensive as sitting in a hospital.

Besides making patients feel anxious and impotent, the "fear of the unknown" distracts patients. A display of skepticism, a sense of distance, or an unwillingness to fully participate in office procedures, even care recommendations, are symptoms of this overlooked dimension of being a new patient. Even staff members, who know that no one has gotten a stroke or been paralyzed by the doctor, can act inappropriately casual, making the patient feel friendless and alone.

Because you're familiar with your office procedures and their rationale, it is easy to lose sight of how a patient feels when encountering what you see as routine. Even if your office staff bends over backward to honor the patient's respect and dignity, patients won't know it until afterwards. Volunteer information in advance to get the maximum patient benefit from your openness and respect for patients.

For example. When you present patients with their admitting paperwork, give them an overview of the first visit protocol.

WELCOME TO THE OFFICE OF DR. SOANDSO

To insure your first visit with us is a pleasant one, here are the procedures you can expect during the next 00 minutes with us:

1. Paperwork: Complete this brief questionnaire to help us get to know you. The doctor will use this information to help formulate your care program.

2. Video: To acquaint you with our office and explain how we help our patients regain their health, most patients see a short 9 minute video.

3. Consultation: You'll meet Dr. SoAndSo, who will review your health history and determine if your's is a chiropractic case. You will be advised of the cost of any office procedures and given a copy of our written financial policies.

4. Examination: Standard physical, orthopedic, neurological, and chiropractic tests will be performed to determine the cause(s) of your problem.

5. X-rays: Necessary views may be taken to visualize the location of any spinal problems, reveal any pathologies, and make your chiropractic care more precise.

6. Correlation: Before proper care can be rendered the doctor will study your examination findings. Later, you'll see your X-rays, review the doctor's findings, and get his specific care recommendations.

7. Adjunctive procedures: The doctor may suggest the application of ice, heat, or the use of some other procedure to help reduce inflammation and make you more comfortable.

8. Future visits: Your first visit is complete. Plan to spend about 00 minutes on your next visit to receive the doctor's report of findings and a chiropractic adjustment. Then, typical visits will usually last only about 00 minutes.

Obviously the specifics would vary from office to office, depending on whether you adjust on the first visit, use any therapy, or perform other procedures. The objective is to give patients a road map of what to expect but most importantly, *why* the procedure is done. Watch new patient rapport improve when you so visibly demonstrate your respect for them.

The same holds true on the patient's second visit in which the report of findings is given and patients usually receive their first adjustment. Using the same style as before, communicate something like this:

WELCOME BACK

Today the doctor will explain the results of your examinations, offer choices for appropriate care, and begin your chiropractic care. Here's what you can expect:

1. Video: You'll see a short video so you can understand your X-rays and the doctor's report and recommendations.

2. Report of findings: You'll see your X-rays and receive a complete report of the examination findings.

3. Treatment plan: The doctor will outline a treatment plan designed for your unique spinal problem and health complaint.

4. Expectations: Based on his or her clinical experience, the doctor will explain your prospects for recovery and what you can do to help speed the healing process.

5. Financial issues: So we can direct all of our attention to your recovery, the financial responsibility for your case will be discussed.

6. Questions: Make sure you fully understand the nature and severity of your condition and what our office will be doing to help you. Ask questions!

7. Adjustments: The doctor will use a carefully directed and controlled pressure to restore the movable bones of your spine to a more normal motion and position. These procedures are called chiropractic adjustments.

8. Adjunctive procedures: If necessary, Dr. SoAndSo may also recommend the application of ice, heat, or the use of other procedures to help reduce inflammation and make you more comfortable.

9. Future visits: Your second visit with us is complete. Future visits will be of a more typical length, usually about 00 minutes.

Explaining your procedures in advance is a way you raise a patient's confidence and self-esteem. When you honor patients and treat them with more respect than they encounter elsewhere in their lives, you create a patient that is more responsive, more responsible, and more likely to refer others. ■

13 WAYS TO
IMPROVE YOUR
YELLOW PAGE AD

When two Phoenix lawyers opened their Legal Clinic in 1976 they felt their approach to providing low cost legal services was a resource their entire community should know about. Invoking the freedom of speech provisions of the United States Constitution, and against the canons of the Arizona State Bar Association, they started advertising their services. The legal battle that ensued, ending up in the United States Supreme Court, ultimately opened the floodgates for all types of licensed professionals to advertise. The result has been an embarrassment to lawyers, dentists, and chiropractors.

This new freedom has invited doctors, lawyers, and other professionals into a domain previously reserved for plumbers and retailers. Besides being a new discipline to master, yellow page advertising is different than any other form of advertising. The approaches suggested by the newspaper classified salesman turned yellow page advertising expert, that worked for transmission specialists and pet stores, don't automatically translate into the health care arena.

Why use the yellow pages? Prospective patients consulting the yellow pages are ready to make a buying decision. "Listing" advertising like the yellow pages is different than direct mail or newspaper advertising. When you're in the yellow pages you're positioned where some prospective patients want to find you. Whoever sees your ad is ready to purchase chiropractic care. They're not deciding *whether* they want a medical doctor or a chiropractic doctor, they're deciding *which* chiropractor. Plus, the yellow pages can help you differentiate your services from other chiropractic offices, educate prospective patients, prequalify the types of patients that you attract, and reduce the anxiety new patients might have about chiropractic.

While I think money spent in the yellow pages could be better spent within the four walls of your clinic, here are some ideas to consider the next time the salesperson from the yellow pages comes begging at your office:

1. Identify your market. Every practitioner has a particular demographic (age, sex, occupation, income, etc.) and psychographic (attitude, values, self-esteem, etc.) that they especially enjoy serving. Why not attract more of the kinds of patients you like? Determine your ideal patient before creating your ad and then write and design your ad to appeal to this distinct market. Just because someone reading your ad has a spine, doesn't automatically make them the type of patient you want!

2. Buy the largest ad you can afford. It's hardly any surprise that research suggests customers tend to call the largest ads first. Whether this is because larger ads are positioned towards the front of the chiropractic section, or that the larger size suggests that your business is more successful, is hard to tell.

Today, with two or more yellow page directories begging for your ad, it's tempting to place an ad in each book. Unfortunately this "divide and conquer" approach dilutes your impact. Instead, poll your current patients. Which directory do they use? Find out and invest the majority of your budget in a single directory.

3. Differentiate your practice. Sadly, many doctors market their practice as if they were offering a commodity like sugar, coffee, or pork bellies. No two practices are alike, even if they use the same examination procedures, X-ray equipment, adjusting technique, and chiropractic brochures. Unlike many retail businesses or large corporate entities, your personality, experience, and specialities are unique factors. While you may be reluctant to boast about your professional accomplishments, explain the way you create a treatment program, or reveal your own health attitudes, these factors can quickly differentiate you and attract patients you'd enjoy serving. Let prospective patients know you're different.

4. Use lots of copy. Unlike newspaper advertising, research by the Lincoln Marketing Group suggest that in the yellow pages "heavy" copy out pulls light copy by 3 to 1. Even in small ads lots of words seems to work better.

Use your copy to differentiate yourself. Avoid copy that restates the obvious or lists services that virtually all chiropractors offer. Put yourself in the shoes of a prospective apprehensive new patient. What would they want to know about you and your office?

Be warned! Your yellow page representative is likely to say, "Looks to me like you have too much copy." Ignore their well-intentioned advice. They are simply applying the same guidance they give the chimney sweep, dog groomer, and the other chiropractors down the street.

5. Remove internal dialogue. Prospective patients reading the yellow pages are probably in pain and have heard stories about chiropractors. They've heard that chiropractors aren't educated, are expensive, and will ask you to come for the rest of their lives. You can take a major step toward better new patient rapport by volunteering information to help dispel these myths. Don't be apologetic! Volunteer information that can serve to put an apprehensive new patient at ease. Your willingness to supply this information can be a very attractive and unique feature of your office.

6. Use a benefit-oriented headline. Headlines serve the same purpose in yellow page advertising as they do in newspaper or magazine advertising; to attract attention. The major difference is that your audience is predisposed to chiropractic. Tailor your headline to the benefits your prospective patient is seeking. What does a new patient seeking chiropractic care in the yellow pages want? Pain relief or wellness care for their children? Probably relief.

7. Include a photograph. Your appearance plays a role in a patient's willingness to trust your recommendations, comply with your recommendations, and even select your office. Do you look friendly? Compassionate? Approachable? Experienced? These are questions that run through the minds of a new patient. If your appearance isn't an asset, either because you look too young or your facial hair projects the image of a "fringe" practitioner, don't include your picture.

If you include a picture of yourself make sure it's big enough! Have a new picture taken and explain to the photographer its end use. Because of the coarse screen used in the yellow pages request a low contrast black and white print for best reproduction.

8. Avoid red ink. With increasing competition, publishers are offering a host of new services, including coupons, "talking yellow pages," and a rainbow of ink colors. Red headlines and blue borders can make sense in a sea of a dozen or more ads with monotone gray ink in the newspaper. However, the color of ink you use in the yellow pages is unlikely to attract more readers than a reassuring headline or volunteering the answers to the most frequently asked questions about chiropractic. Instead, spend your money on a larger ad.

9. Monitor your results. Every dime of your marketing efforts should be held accountable. You'll never know if these ideas really work or what to do differently next year, unless you keep track of the source of your new patients.

Create a simple form so the staff member who answers the phone can ask them how they found out about your office. Asking them while they are still on the phone will render more accurate information than later when they're in your office. For further confirmation, repeat the question on your new patient admitting form, including medium such as television, direct mail, or others you may not even use. Plot the source of your new patients each month on a graph. It will make decisions about next year's advertising easier to make and justify.

10. Include a map. Research by the National Research Group in Lincoln, Nebraska suggest those who use the yellow pages for health care services have lived in the community less than five years. These newcomers may need some help in finding your office. If space doesn't allow a map, describe your location in the context of a major intersection, popular retail store, or local landmark.

11. Have a call to action. Ask for some type of commitment. While "asking for the order" may make you uneasy, look at your request from a patient's point of view. You're not pandering to the general public, you're talking to someone who probably desperately needs your help.

In fact, they're so apprehensive they've waited for weeks or months before opening the yellow pages. Help them over their fear by encouraging them to take the first step towards relief and better health.

12. Get your ad professionally produced. Resist the temptation of delegating the design of your ad to one of the "artists" that work for the directory publisher! Hire a professional. Considering the investment you're about to make, make sure your ad projects a contemporary image and doesn't look like the upholstery shop ad down the street.

Consult the yellow pages and look under Graphic Designer for a commercial artist that can help you. Set some appointments to review their portfolios and discuss your design needs. Maybe have him or her rework your letterhead and business card at the same time.

13. Avoid the pack. Many of these ideas run counter to what your yellow page salesperson and even your graphic designer is used to. Everyone will attempt to talk you out of making waves. It takes courage to stand out. But isn't that one of the reasons you chose chiropractic?

Yellow page advertising will always be more an art than a science. Most businesses admit that half of their advertising doesn't work. They just don't know which half! ■

TURNING JUNK
INTO JEWELS

A 1988 survey revealed that 27% of the chiropractic profession uses some type of periodic newsletter mailing. Marketing specialists who claim newsletters don't work or are a waste of time, either have unreasonable expectations or entertain a short-term vision of the doctor/patient relationship. Few newsletters will produce patients the day after they are mailed. Instead, most of the ones I've seen ignore the fundamental rules of written communication, impairing their effectiveness. This is especially important if you consider the fact that most of your patients see your newsletter as just more junk mail!

What's the purpose of a newsletter? Without a clearly defined purpose, a newsletter can seem like a lot of extra work, a nuisance, and an unnecessary expense. With a definite (and measurable goal) it can be an exciting opportunity. A newsletter can inform and inspire your patients and serve as a vehicle for reminding them of their relationship with your office. It should be easy to create and accountable in its performance. If it isn't, you'll create your first issue in a burst of enthusiasm and the well known benefits of repetition will be lost.

Use your newsletter as a way of educating your patients. While this is an honorable goal, be reminded of the narrow appeal of public broadcasting! Reading requires more work than just passively watching television—your newsletter should be highly visual and entertaining too. Not necessarily every article, but make an effort to entertain as you educate. People learn more while they're laughing than when they're bored.

Others see their newsletter as a way to motivate patients, affirming their decision to seek chiropractic care. They include testimonials of patients bringing their children and newborns to the office. They share examples of patients who have chosen rehabilitative or maintenance care so new patients will realize there is more to chiropractic than pain relief.

Ideally a newsletter offers a variety of short educational, entertaining, and motivational articles that are interesting and to the point. But on what subjects?

Chiropractic of course! But lest patients perceive your newsletter as propaganda, consider taking a broader, wellness approach and include a wide range of subjects such as dental health, nutrition, exercise, mental health, pediatrics, and others. Help patients get a holistic picture of wellness health care. Each issue should have something from the doctor that helps reveal the doctor's personality, philosophy, or expertise. Similarly, consider short biographical sketches about yourself and other staff members. It's a great way to add some humor, human interest, and reveal interesting facts that may not come up in conversation in the adjusting room or at the front desk. Give patients a way to build a deeper relationship with the office than Wednesdays at 4:15 P.M.

How long should the articles be? With all the books about how to be a "one minute" just about anything, keep your articles and stories down to one minute or less. Most of us read about 200-300 words per minute at the eighth grade level (*People* magazine or *Reader's Digest*). But more than that, it's better to have five, 100 word articles, than two, 250 word articles. You want as many "entry points" as possible, especially on the front page of a multi-page newsletter. With more entry points you have a better chance of capturing your reader. Otherwise, if the reader isn't captivated by your featured "cover story," he or she may be less likely to continue reading.

As you edit and shorten the articles ask yourself the "So what?" question—so your audience won't! How will a patient or potential patient benefit from reading each article? Will you share a little known fact? Will your information enhance their lives? What difference will it make? These are not difficult questions for your articles to answer, especially when working in chiropractic. Keep them in mind so your newsletter is valued, read, kept, shared with a friend, or used as a referral tool.

How frequently should you publish your newsletter? For some offices it's so traumatic or time-consuming it's done quarterly. Unfortunately with the objectives mentioned above, combined with the average length of care, quarterly may be too infrequent. Many patients may begin and drop out of care between issues! Instead, simplify your newsletter to a single-sided page that can be mailed monthly. Always have at least one photograph or illustration (with a caption!) on the cover.

You may want to avoid information that is dated, like birthdays and references to the season. Number the issues, but don't date them. Then, when you print your newsletter, print up a couple hundred extras and save them on the shelf. When new patients begin care send them a newsletter once a week until you're caught up with the current monthly-produced issue. It's during this early stage of their care that they are most interested in chiropractic, so nurture them with frequent mailings using back issues.

Who should you mail it to? Obviously active and inactive patients. And with the stigma of junk mail removed by short, benefit-oriented writing, send it to as many others as your budget allows. Start your non-patient mailing list with vendors, suppliers, and others who come into contact with your office on a business level. Consider other health care providers too, especially others in your community who provide wellness health care services who might serve as a source of referrals. And finally, if your budget permits, consider a bulk mailing to a 3-5 mile radius of your office. This is the typical geographical area your office serves and these households represent a major source of new patients.

How do you get your newsletter produced? Until recently there were few choices for the actual production of a newsletter. You could send the material to a typesetter or have your printer get it typeset, or use a typewriter to set the type yourself. Advances in computer technology have added another choice: desktop publishing.

Desktop publishing is a term used to broadly describe a computer program that hyphenates words, arranges copy into columns, offers a choice of typestyles, and does other typographical chores which are then printed on a laser printer. The near typeset quality and speed make desktop publishing a very attractive alternative to organizations that would normally use typesetting services for reports, presentations, newsletters, and other important internal documents.

Today, many "quick print" types of print shops are adding desktop publishing capabilities. Because the equipment is getting simpler to operate, some printers allow customers to enter and compose their material after a brief training session. Others have an operator who enters and formats the material for clients. Either way, this new technology has significantly lowered the price of producing a newsletter and, as expected, resulted in an explosion of newsletters, sales literature, and junk mail flooding our homes and businesses. In this environment, good design and customer benefit-oriented content become even more important.

After your articles are written and their order determined, the desktop publishing program prints an entire page of text at one time. Needless to say, proof your material at every stage along the way for typographical or grammatical errors. Typos are the constant frustration of any publisher. Yet invariably a few slip by. Typos are impossible to correct after you print and send your newsletter. Use the carpenter's adage, "Measure twice, cut once." Interestingly, the best way to proof for typographical errors is to read the document backwards. Since you won't be distracted by the meaning of the individual words, spelling problems are easier to spot. Another helpful test is to have someone unfamiliar with the material read it aloud.

How do you select a printer? First you must know the scope of work. How many pages will your newsletter be? What size of paper? What kind of paper—coated or uncoated, colored or white? How many do you intend to print? One color or two color or more? Being able to supply this information over the telephone can help you identify printers in your area who are comfortable with your size of project. Some printers cannot afford to tie up their presses unless you're printing thousands of copies. Other printers get nervous with runs greater than 500. The challenge is to find a printer with the quality, price, and interest to serve your needs. When you've found two or three printers that seem to meet this criteria, discuss the project in more detail and ask for written bids. Prices from printers offering similar quality can vary depending upon how busy they are.

Before actually printing your newsletter, consult with a direct mailing facility to make sure your design will meet postal regulations. If the size of your mailing is large enough (more than 200 pieces) most facilities will encourage you to print their bulk mail permit number on your newsletter. This lowers the postage costs and simplifies mail room preparation. These same companies usually have their own mailing lists of residents in your community sorted by zip code. If you intend to mail to a geographical area around your office they can probably help with that too, so you'll know how many copies of your newsletter to print.

Your newsletter should reflect the tone of your office and be in step with today's graphic standards. The days in which a typewritten mimeographed page would work are long gone. Today, with so many things begging for our attention, a newsletter should be short, to the point, very visual, and enhance the reader's perception of his or her health and well being. When it does, you've transformed a piece of junk mail into a strategic practice growth tool. ■

WANTING WHAT
THEY NEED

Every weekend there is an interesting phenomenon that occurs in neighborhoods around the country. Garage sales. Usually once a year or so, closets are cleaned out, the basement is inspected, and the clutter in the garage is emptied of things no longer wanted. The gasoline powered weed eater. The bowling ball no longer used. Clothing that no longer fits. Dishes, knick-knacks, and the now abandoned fish aquarium. The prices applied by masking tape are a bargain. Perfectly good and functioning items for sometimes less than 10 percent of what they were originally purchased for. It's a good example of what happens when needs change, people grow, or they have confused what they want with what they need.

I bet many of the items at a garage sale were purchased on impulse or without a clear understanding of the responsibilities or the maintenance needed. Other items may have simply been outgrown. When it was purchased, virtually every item was wanted. "I just gotta have that new-improved-super-charged" whatever. This type of behavior is most obvious in children who go from one thing to another, wanting this and wanting that. These discarded things are rarely "needed" but they are desired (wanted) at the time. Then times change.

There is a tendency among those who are the most philosophically dogmatic in chiropractic to look down upon patients who merely want pain relief. "I don't treat symptoms," they say smugly as their nose tilts ever so slightly towards heaven. "What the patient *needs* is spinal rehabilitation and lifetime maintenance care," they rationalize to themselves. But what the patient wants is pain relief. "I don't treat symptoms," deadpans the doctor. "Medical doctors treat symptoms, I treat the cause." It seems so clear to the doctor. And while the doctor is able to maintain his or her philosophical "purity," patients don't get it.

When I was doing work for Compassion International, a Christian child sponsorship organization, I saw first hand, the importance of recognizing the difference between wants and needs.

In the Third World, poverty is one of the greatest challenges, particularly in the "mega cities" of Mexico City, Manila, Hong Kong, and countless others. In these and other cities, I have seen human squalor and hopelessness that will tug at my consciousness for the rest of my life. Millions have fled beautiful, quiet rural settings for the bright lights and opportunities of the city. What they find is something vastly different. Without education and training, and with their life savings exhausted, they must take up residence in one of the many slums and cardboard shanty towns of the sprawling city. Lacking the resources to return to their families in the country, they become trapped. The objective of Compassion International and many other child sponsorship organizations, is to provide educational opportunities for the children who are hit hardest by poverty so they can eventually escape the "cycle of poverty" imprisoning their parents.

Those in this horrible existence need food, shelter, and a job. But that's not necessarily what they *want*. They want a television. And the things advertised on it. That was one of the most striking impressions I have of one of the worst slums in Manila. Amongst the leaking tin roofs and mud floors in hut after rickety hut, was the glowing phosphorous of television screens. In the comfort of our plush homes and profitable offices we could say that they shouldn't want television. What they need is a good education and to work hard so they can pull themselves up by their bootstraps. Yet, in the midst of this human suffering and starvation is a most extreme example of how wants overpower and obscure needs.

At the most extreme survival level one's wants and needs are usually identical. It's not until we have a disposable income that these two concepts diverge and the implications of our choices become more complicated. Suddenly we want several TVs, cars, boats, the latest high tech tennis shoes, and everything we see in the stores. As our income rises so does our spending. Our self-esteem often becomes entrapped by the things we surround ourselves with.

Parents who really love their children give them what they need. We give them vegetables at dinner, even though they want sweets. We enforce a reasonable bedtime, even though they want to fall asleep in front of the TV. We insist they brush their teeth, even though they may not want to.

When you attempt to give patients what they need before giving them what they want, you're treating them like children. And they resent it. These good intentions often backfire, creating an exclusivity about your practice, counterproductive to your calling to help humanity. Why not acknowledge their lack of understanding and accept the opportunity to educate them and increase their awareness? Why penalize them or deny them what they want simply because they should know better?

When this "healthier-than-thou" attitude is exhibited in religious circles, we see the do-gooder who cannot lower himself to rub shoulders with the unclean sinners. This obstructs evangelism. Those smug in their faith can rest assured that their own fragile beliefs won't be tested by encounters with those who ask tough questions or don't understand the religious jargon.

Sadly, medicine has always been quick to give patients what they want. Want pain relief? Take this. Want to avoid polio? Ingest this. That gall bladder of yours giving you trouble? We better take it out. A little depressed? Change your blood chemistry with these. And on it goes. This trains patients that "solutions" come from outside the body. Remember, this attitude is the "pre-existing condition" practically every new patient enters your office with. It doesn't make them less deserving of chiropractic, nor does it preclude them growing in their understanding of health under your tutelage. Wishful thinking or one more chiropractic philosophy seminar isn't going to change this reality.

When patients enter your office and reveal that their health awareness doesn't extend beyond getting out of pain, you have several choices.

Refer out. You can send them down the street because you "don't do pain relief only" chiropractic. This selfish attitude denies chiropractic to patients who have not yet progressed to your high standards. Since patients with this attitude require more work and may demean your role as a doctor and relegate your clinical skills to just a drugless form of pain relief, it's tempting to make them feel unwelcome. They are usually skeptical and not a lot of fun to be around. They are merely the product of a culture that has been weaned on a medical approach to life. Sure, send them down the street until they "grow up." Make them feel like a loser.

Accept with reservations. They have completed your admission form indicating they want relief only. You can accept their limited vision, attempt to normalize their spinal biomechanics, and allow them to dismiss themselves. Ignore the personality distortion their pain is causing. Overlook the fact they might not understand the implications of words like rehabilitation or spinal reconstruction. Invite them in to get a taste of chiropractic and keep your expectations low. Educate them so they have a chance to grow in the understanding of what you really do. Acquire the trust and lay a foundation on which you or some other chiropractic doctor can build on in the future. Instead of fixing your eye on the center field fence, just try getting on base.

Accept and educate. Embracing chiropractic is the result of making many small decisions, culminating in the courage to call your office. And while you can complain about the health attitudes of the general population, casting dispersions on their incompetence and shortsighted-ness from your chiropractic ivory tower is easy, it's wrong. Honor them by accepting their limited view of health and consider it an opportunity while they are within your sphere of influence to educate and enlarge their appreciation of true health.

Waiting for a sufficient number of patients who are "good enough" or who are available for true health is a slow way to grow your practice and influence your community. If you recognize that the understanding and practice of good spinal hygiene is a learning process, commit to helping anyone who wanders into your office. That doesn't mean they'll "get it," however you'll be sowing seeds that you may reap months or years from now. What's the hurry?

Growing a patient's understanding of health requires confrontation, courage, and patience. Clearly it requires clinical confidence and excellent communication skills. Realize that you can't wait for the made-for-TV movies, a *20/20* documentary, or the medical-oriented media to change and nurture proper health attitudes. If you watch a few Saturday morning cartoons you'll see that another generation may already be lost to a shortsighted vision of health. If there is going to be a change, it's going to happen in offices like yours, one patient at a time. It will mean accepting patients on their terms, giving them what they want and earning the right to give them what they need. ■

METAPHORICALLY
SPEAKING

Since better communication results in a better practice and communication skills are not innate, but a learned behavior, improving one's ability to communicate can make a dramatic difference in your practice. An increasing number of communication tools and resources are being presented to chiropractors from within and from without the profession. Being aware of these techniques and consistently implementing them are two different things!

Neuro-Linguistic Programming (NLP) has received considerable attention in the last five or six years. Anthony Robbins and his famous "firewalk" are perhaps the most visible examples of the popularization and acceptance of this communication technology. His bestselling book, *Unlimited Power*, describes some of the techniques of mirroring, pacing, swish patterns, anchoring, and others. These and related communication insights recognize how the brain works and organizes the presentation of information in a language more likely to be understood. Doctors and staff can take cues from a patient's language and determine whether they are more likely to be receptive to visual, aural, or kinesthetically encoded messages. The rationale here is that if a patient favors information presented in a visual format (the majority of today's TV-weaned public) and you present information to them orally at the report of findings, the impact and understanding of your message is diminished.

A slightly different twist is offered by author Bert Decker in his book,

You've Got To Be Believed To Be Heard. He suggests that all communication with others is filtered through the primitive part of our brains, which decides whether we believe the person sending the message. Decker emphasizes that these decisions are based on the non-verbal portion of the message. This picks up the theme expressed by Marshall McLuhan that "the media is the message." That is, *how* you communicate is often more important than *what* you communicate.

Doctors with an analytical bent or defensive attitude are often unaware of this and tend to place an inordinate amount of attention in explaining a patient's range of motion in degrees or other measurable details. In fact, some doctors revel in this data, and report it in so much detail, they fail to notice the glazed look in their patient's eyes.

Facts and figures rarely convince anyone other than accountants and scientists. Decker suggests that we make all of our decisions emotionally and then justify or rationalize them with facts. For example, if you were a patient emerging from relief care, which reasons would be more motivational, the emotional impact of being told you would be able to pick up your grandchildren in your old age or that continued care is important to slow the degeneration process? Would you rather gain a better golf swing or improve a kyphotic curve by 10 degrees? If patients were rational, they'd make the right decisions based on your objective clinical findings. Instead, their compliance is often shaped by a much more subtle factor—how you communicate.

It takes more than just converting data into usable, real-world information that makes a difference. It's the non-verbal dimension that sabotages many doctors and staff members. Patients desperately want to know that they're in the right place and that they've selected a practitioner that can help. Patients must receive unconscious assurances from the doctor's body language that he or she has the personal confidence and experience to help the patient. Patients are sensitive and may correctly or incorrectly detect or interpret a pause, a glance away, a shifting in your chair, or other subtle movement or posture as a lack of assurance, undermining their compliance and even the healing process! A patient's hope or trust in your recommendations can be dashed by the smallest detail that suggests incongruency or a mixed message. Doctors must broadcast similar messages at all levels, conscious and unconscious. Doctors who practice fearlessly exude verbal and nonverbal confidence that reassures apprehensive patients and enhances their compliance and prospects for recovery. This suggests that whether you're a 20-year chiropractic veteran or just venturing into practice, the first person the doctor has to convince—is the doctor!

Along with communicating a high level of confidence in your chiropractic skills through your body language, it's important to use the most effective words and phrases. Taking a cue from the best communicators this planet has ever seen, doctors should be using more metaphors. The most effective communicators have always used metaphors, parables, short stories, fairy tales and similar devices when communicating new ideas to the masses. A metaphor is a way of saying, "this new thing" is like this "old thing." In fact, using the word "like" is almost a guarantee that the concept that follows is metaphorical. By associating a new idea with one already commonly understood helps patients accept it. It not only reduces misunderstandings but it also can equip patients with a ready way of telling others about chiropractic or any other new idea. Using metaphors can improve referrals.

After years of schooling and clinical experience it's easy to take many chiropractic words and concepts for granted. It's easy to forget that most new patients haven't the foggiest idea what an adjustment, subluxation, or nerve interference is. Overlook this, building your verbal presentation on these words without a proper explanation, and patients don't "get it." Metaphors can help new patients understand these new ideas. Certainly this isn't a conclusive list, but here are some metaphors that many effective communicators use with their patients:

Subluxation: Describe a kink in a hose or what an auto accident does to freeway traffic.

Adjustment: The process of aligning the front end of a car, tuning in a radio station, or the fine tuning of a mechanical device.

Spinal Kinesiopathology: Orthodontics is a good way of describing the affect of abnormal motion or position of spinal bones. Adjustments can be likened to braces on teeth (bones). I like the notion of pelvic tilt causing problems to the spine up above like the settling of a house foundation causing cracks in the walls.

Neuropathophysiology: The concept of nervous system malfunction is like television when your cable goes out—you can see the picture, but there's a lot of static. The dimmer switch works well too. In fact, make sure the room you give your report of findings has a dimmer switch so you could illustrate it during your report.

Myopathology: The scar tissue that changes the elasticity of the muscle is like gristle in an inexpensive steak. Muscles adapt and get used to supporting the spine improperly, like trying to change your hair part. A tug of war. The stronger team (muscles attached to the spinous process) causes the bone to rotate.

Histopathology: A bruise, black eye, sunburn, blister, and jelly-filled donut can be quite effective.

Pathophysiology: I like the mineral deposits in a cave (stalactites and stalagmites) because it suggests that given enough time the bones will fuse together. Barnacles on a rock is an easy way to show the idea of bone spurs. Or lighten up your explanation by suggesting it's like having your house remodeled by an amateur carpenter. The concept of tooth decay works well too. Decay is simpler and probably carries more impact than the word degeneration.

After years of school, making countless drawings of the spine and having a love of its physiology, it's easy to forget that patients have difficulty understanding your chiropractic perspective. Without a complete understanding, patients lack the basis for properly respecting your clinical skills. More significant to those interested in growing their practice, it makes it difficult for patients to explain chiropractic to others.

Improving one's communication skills can do more to improve a practice than all the technique workshops in the world. Using metaphors in your patient communications is like the difference between earphones and speakers. Earphones are more personal and only one person can hear at a time. Like metaphors, a set of loud speakers allow more people to hear your message. Metaphorically, you'll know they "got it" when you see the light bulb go on above their heads. ■

DOCTOR OR MECHANIC?

Having entered the chiropractic profession by helping create patient education tools for Renaissance International in the early 1980s, I sometimes forget there are chiropractors who do not educate their patients. At a recent chiropractic convention I asked some of the doctors why they didn't educate their patients. The excuses and rationalizations surprised me.

"My patients are uneducable." Oh really? How did he attract an entire practice of learning disabled patients? Further questioning revealed he had a practice that was largely worker's compensation and personal injury cases of Hispanic descent. "Their care is paid for by insurance and they don't want to learn anything about chiropractic. They want to get fixed and back to work," he said flashing his gold capped teeth.

Detroit has made driving a car so easy you don't even have to know how it works to use one. One pedal is for go and one pedal is for stop. Use the big round thing to turn to the right or left. You don't need to know how an internal combustion engine works, how an automatic transmission works, or how the turbo works. Yet, drivers who know how these devices work, find their cars get better gas mileage, last longer, and require fewer repairs.

It's the same with basic physiology. Patients who understand how their bodies work are less likely to get sick and when they do, get well faster. Ask your most disinterested patients, if they'd be interested in learning some ways of saving money, getting well faster, and preventing their problems from recurring in the future? Watch their eyes light up!

If patients don't care, it's because the doctor isn't sensitive or creative enough to find an entry point. Remember the best teachers you had in school? They were the ones that made learning relevant. The less effective teachers were too philosophical, egotistical, not practical, or so uninterested in the material themselves they were unable to make it interesting for their students. How are you making chiropractic fun and interesting for your patients?

"It's too much work." That's what one tired doctor said. Apparently at one time he had recognized the need, but it became too labor intensive or the rejection from patients (because it wasn't relevant) wore him out. Without experiencing the rewards of your efforts, it *can* seem like work. Hauling out the lecture charts, begging patients to attend, shoving brochures at patients, and all the other means can test anyone's patience.

I have an uncle who is a dry wheat farmer in Colorado. He cultivates the ground, plants the seed, waits for the seed to germinate and green buds to poke up through the soil. In the early part of spring that can take weeks. But that's just the start. How about the insects, diseases, lack of rain, damaging hail, and all the other challenges? If you require instant gratification, don't become a farmer.

Patient education is a lot like seed planting. The difference of course is that you don't know when or if your efforts will germinate. If you want to avoid disappointment, simply don't plant any seeds.

"Not enough time." This is the "I'm-so-busy-putting-out-fires-I-don't-have-time-for-fire-prevention" school of thought. This type of practice makes doctors feel important and valuable. Because it is largely a practice of symptomatic patients who respond to the pain relief aspect of chiropractic, the doctor can rest assured that "chiropractic works." This medical approach to chiropractic (symptom relief only) fits the insurance model perfectly, as patients discontinue care when they feel better. Forget about the soft tissue and underlying muscle damage that predisposes them to a relapse. Ignore the value of some type of on-going maintenance or wellness care like you enjoy! After all, you're running a pain clinic.

What are these doctors going to do when their highly-leveraged lifestyles and cluttered insurance departments regularly encounter $1000 deductibles or patients without insurance? "By then, the nationalized health plan like Canada's will be in effect," they respond smugly. How chiropractic will fair is anyone's guess. However, if you think Canadian chiropractors are delighted with the 12 visits or 22 visits doled out in the various provinces, you need to meet a few of them. Better yet, talk to a few chiropractors in Oregon, Colorado, and Minnesota who, in the early 1990s, felt the cost-containment moods of their legislatures. This is a wake up call! Changes are coming. Big changes.

"I already educate my patients." I was intrigued by his confidence and Mr. KnowItAll attitude. Prepared to learn some new technique or gain some fresh insight into patient education I asked him about his various approaches. "It's basically at the report of findings," he said without blinking. "I show them their X-rays, explain my examination findings, and make my recommendations for care."

I was caught off guard, expecting some systematized patient dialogue, innovative brochure presentation, or "topic of the day" program he was using. "So you feel that your report pretty much acquaints patients with what they need to know?" I asked regaining my composure.

"It seems to be working," he smiled.

"Great," I said.

This is the "magic pill" school of thought in which patients are expected to abandon a lifetime of medical/germ theory/aspirin-popping orientation after a spellbinding 15-minute patter in front of the X-ray view box!

If you're feeling confident of your current patient education efforts, give some of your brightest pupils a pop quiz:

1. Would you rather feel good or be healthy?

2. If you throw up after eating food that has been improperly prepared are you sick or are you well?

3. Why is it that when 10 people are exposed to a cold virus only a few people get one?

4. What controls the function of every cell, tissue, and organ of your body?

5. Describe what a chiropractic adjustment is and what it does.

Offices that invest heavily in patient education tools and techniques do so because they understand the huge return on their investment. Here are some reasons why patient education pays off in today's most successful practices:

Faster healing: Researchers in a Minneapolis hospital studied two groups of cardiac patients. To one group they volunteered a complete explanation of the procedure and discussed the possible post-operative reactions. To the other they took a more traditional approach, only answering questions asked by the patients. The result? The "educated" patients recovered twice as fast.

Better compliance: Getting patients to do the right thing to participate in their own recovery is enhanced through patient education. Blindly following "doctor's orders" is no longer the standard protocol. Today, patients want to know *why* it takes more than one visit, *why* it feels sore after their first adjustment, *why* they should bring in their children, and answers to countless other "why?" questions.

More referrals: The most enjoyable patients to serve are those your current patients refer to your office. When your current patients vouch for you, new patients are less critical and skeptical. Your patients could generate even more referrals if they could more accurately describe what chiropractic is, and adequately defend the value of their chiropractic lifestyle. If your patients can't explain to a friend why someone with headaches or some type of systemic problem might benefit from chiropractic care, they won't.

Less stress: When patients understand their chiropractic care there is less confrontation and fewer inappropriate questions. This allows staff members to better choreograph patient flow and tend to the interpersonal and non-clinical needs of your patients. When patients have a clear understanding as to why they are in the office, there is a genuine sense of family that makes coming to the office a real joy.

More respect: Education gives your patients a greater appreciation for the skill required to be a chiropractor. Without proper education patients are likely to devalue the importance of the adjustment and to assume that all patients receive identical care. "Something so repetitive and quickly rendered must not be very difficult," reasons the patient. Combine this with the word on the street that chiropractors are poorly educated and you have a practice in which patients have little more respect for the doctor than they do for their barber or car mechanic. *Educated patients hold chiropractic doctors in higher esteem than uneducated patients.*

More families: Parents who understand chiropractic are more likely to bring the rest of the family in for care. Parents who understand chiropractic are more likely to bring their newborns in for a chiropractic check up. Often these families show up together, get adjusted together, and make for a very efficient office visit. Measure how well you're educating your patients, by counting the number of children receiving care in your practice. Few 6 year olds will call your office for a free spinal exam! Only educated parents who trust you will bring their children in for care.

More wellness patients: Educated patients are more likely to continue with some type of maintenance care. These are fun patients to be around because they recognize the value of something you've given your life for. These are generally cash-paying patients who provide a stabilizing influence at a time when insurance deductibles are rising. Better still, educated maintenance patients can schedule their visits around your vacations and long weekends with your family. Patient education allows you to have a life.

More chiropractors: Educated patients are more likely to see the career path represented by chiropractic and become chiropractors themselves. I can always tell how well a doctor educates his or her patients by how many patients they have sent to chiropractic college. Patients who have not been educated can't get excited about your profession unless they simply envy your house, your car, or flashy jewelry. Patient education ensures that there will always be enough chiropractors to respond to the increasing demand for chiropractic.

Patients do what they do, because they think like they think. Changing the way they think is a major responsibility of doctors and staff. Not just because it's the right thing to do, but because improving a patient's spinal biomechanics without educating them, ignores the most potent part of their nervous system—the brain. This important part of the nervous system controls patient compliance, retention, referrals, and the less statistically measurable aspects of perception, respect, and trust. Ultimately it is the condition of this organ that will decide if they are seeing a doctor or merely a spine mechanic. ■

POWER WORDS

On a recent flight, the cabin attendant given the responsibility to present the safety monologue while the others pantomimed in the aisle, dropped all the "ing" endings to her words. The result was an uneducated sounding "hick" whose "wannas" and "gonnas" did little to reassure me of her proficiency or experience. Whether we like it or not, our vocabulary, grammar, and pronunciation reveals a lot about us. During those first few minutes after meeting someone new, we quickly judge that person by his or her appearance and ability to communicate.

The ability to express ourselves by using the right words is essential to our success. Some suggest that our vocabularies stop growing in our early 20s. If we cannot express ourselves with accuracy and clarity, we diminish our ability to connect and make an impact with those around us. This is especially true in the doctor/patient relationship. If you depend on words to help your patients "get it" then it's important to use the words that are more likely to generate patient response and avoid those that are ambiguous or diminish the impact of your message.

I've heard certain words crop up again and again as I've eavesdropped on the reports of findings of effective doctors and listened to the tableside discussions of those with good compliance and patient follow-through. Whether they've learned to use these words by trial and error or from attending a lifetime of chiropractic seminars is unimportant. Here are some words they use that seem to enhance the likelihood of producing better patient rapport:

Relief: This is what most patients want. Notice that this word is used extensively in analgesic advertising. It is simple and direct. It can be used without implying a cure and it gets to the heart of what prompted most patients to consult your office in the first place. This doesn't imply that relief is all they need, but it's what they want. "Mrs. Jones, we're going to work together and do everything we can to help you get the relief you want."

Choke: I've come to favor this word over the word "pinch" for explaining the nerve physiology resulting from aberrant spinal bio-mechanics. Remember when Special K breakfast cereal used to advertise about "pinching an inch?" Pinching seems less harmful, even frivolous, when compared with choking. If you've ever seen someone choking in a restaurant, you know what I mean! It's scary. It is loaded with much more serious connotations than a pinch. "The most serious aspect of this problem is that the nerves that run down your leg are being choked as they exit the spinal cord here and here."

Patch: This is an especially powerful way to describe a less desirable form of care that simply addresses the symptoms of a patient's presenting complaint. The word conjures up chronic potholes in the street that require constant attention. Who would want to "patch up" their spinal problem when instead they could rehabilitate or optimize their spine? "At this point in my report of findings I always ask my patients whether they want a patch job or to have the problem truly fixed. What type of care are you interested in?"

Relapse: I don't know why this word isn't used more frequently in chiropractic. Ask any doctor with at least a year of clinical experience what happens to the patient's problem if all they receive is symptomatic care and immediately drop out: their problem comes back. Not 10% of the time. Not 50% of the time. Almost 100% of the time! And prime time soap operas have made the word relapse especially laden with meaning. No one wants a relapse because conventional wisdom suggests it's usually worse and often preventable. "Remember, how long you decided to benefit from chiropractic care is always up to you. However, based on the last seven years of my clinical practice I've noticed that patients who drop out as soon as they feel better are more likely to suffer a relapse."

Decay: You may know it as Subluxation Degeneration but it communicates more impact to refer to it spinal decay. When dentists stopped calling them tooth carries and started calling it tooth decay there was a significant surge in preventive dental care. Even kids can understand what spinal decay must be like! "We only know of two ways to slow or stop this relentless process of spinal decay."

Hope: With the unusually high success rate that chiropractic enjoys, it's sometimes easy to forget how powerful this word (and emotion) is in the healing process. Too many patients show up in a chiropractic office without hope—you are their last resort. Many have been told they will have to learn to live with the pain and still others have been told it's all in their heads. If it's appropriate, give patients reason to be hopeful. The best doctors tap in to this fundamental force of human nature. "Because of your age, condition, and lifestyle I think you have every right to be hopeful."

Results: This is a powerful word for the bottom-line "show-me" attitude that many patients have when they enter your office. There is a directness and no-nonsense attitude projected when using this word. This businesslike word talks a language patients understand—it's what they're paying money for. While it's true that patients expect results, the patient is often more supportive of your efforts and the time required to achieve them when you acknowledge their purpose for seeking care in your office. "We've gotten excellent results with many patients with problems just like yours."

There's nothing magical about any of these words. Using them doesn't cause patients to submit to your every command. They are just simple one and two syllable words that patients understand and seem to respond to. Because doctors who frequently use these types of words appreciate their true meaning and impact, their communication is congruent and believable. Simply scripting them or peppering your conversations with them reduce their impact. These or any other words have power only because of the power behind the doctor's convictions.

"I hope you get the relief and results you deserve, and avoid a relapse

of patching decayed patient conversations that choke their understanding!"

See what I mean? ■

THE LANGUAGE OF CHIROPRACTIC

Words are so pitiful. Communication specialists suggest that more than 90% of the message we send to others is non-verbal. Compared to body language, inflection, energy level, eye movement, and appearance, words are nickels and dimes in the million dollar world of effective communication.

Those most anxious for the most effective recall "script" are often disappointed. "What should I say when the patient says so and so?" A scripted life would be predictable and we could fool ourselves into believing we were in control. Words are extremely ineffective when it comes to communicating at the most meaningful level.

We are visual animals. We obtain most of the information about the world around us through our eyes. Witness the clichés, "Seeing is believing" or "A picture is worth a thousand words" or "I'll believe it when I see it." "Look out!" *See* what I mean? Our language is amply seasoned with a visual orientation.

Granted it is usually a "feeling" that prompts patients to consult your office, but what does chiropractic "look" like to your patients. Are you using visuals to communicate the full nature and severity of their condition? Are you using pictures to explain the relationship between the patient, the patient's insurance carrier, and the doctor? Are you using highly-visual terms to make your recommendations memorable? Or do you numb them with the most expedient and least effective communication commodity, words?

In the offices I've consulted, the doctors' personal and professional success seems related to their level of communication skills. Poor communicators seem to have less effective practices than excellent communicators. Poor communicators have less fulfilling careers than excellent communicators. In fact, I've seen excellent communication skills (verbal and non-verbal) make up for less than astounding adjusting techniques, poor management abilities, and ineffective office procedures. When the chiropractic message is projected through appropriate words, pictures, and congruent body language, patients are more likely to "get it." When patients understand chiropractic, they are empowered to defend their chiropractic decision to others outside the office. When patients more completely understand the chiropractic story, referrals are an obvious by-product. When staff members can visualize the "big idea," telephone scripts become almost unnecessary. When you see the big picture, it's pictures that make the difference.

The ability to communicate in a more effective visual way, has little to do with chiropractic. It's part of a repertoire of interpersonal skills related to the ability to socialize, anticipate the needs of the others, and create meaningful relationships. It is often a reflection of one's self-esteem. Those with high self-esteem seem to be better communi-cators. Those with low self-esteem figure no one's interested or are afraid of taking what might be an unpopular stand. The resulting patient perception is the doctor's lack of conviction and confidence, undermining the patient's trust, patience, willingness to comply, and ultimately the healing process itself. Effective communication is a crucial aspect of a successful practice—especially something as misunderstood as chiropractic.

Getting away from words for a moment, what are other non-verbal ways of communicating? Before exploring the visual opportunities for more effective communication, consider some of the other sensory inputs such as smell, taste, and touch. How are you using olfactory stimulation in your office? What does your office smell like? The hydroculator? The X-ray film processor? The cigarette smoke clinging to the C.A.'s hair? The billiard room next door to your office? The last patient?

Our culture tends to downplay the role of smell. Go to any Third World marketplace and drink in the aroma of freshly ground spices, ripe fruits, and colorful vegetables. Our supermarkets protect everything in plastic wrap, insulating us from an important constituent in the buying decision—smell.

In 1986 a popular general interest magazine conducted a remarkable "scratch and sniff" study among its readers to determine some of the psychological effects of different aromas. They discovered the most stressful aromas were those associated with mint; spearmint, wintergreen, etc. The most restful were vanilla and apple pie. Virtually anyone who has tried to sell their home has been told to bake bread or a pie before the big open house. The objective is to associate a positive sensory input with the business at hand—selling the house.

Ever catch a whiff of perfume or cologne in a large crowd that you remember from high school? The memories come flooding back in torrents you can't control. Our brains are wired in such a way that aroma is a powerful mnemonic device. Offices that enjoy trying new things have begun adding aroma to the adjusting table head rest paper! The aroma applied to the edges of the head rest paper become associated with the chiropractic adjustment. Vanilla. Orange. Butterscotch. "May I go into the 'chocolate room' for my adjustment today?" Mix it up. Have some fun. Give patients something to look forward to! Outside your office, what do you think patients will think of every time they have vanilla ice cream? Chiropractic of course!

Apply the same idea to sound. What does your office sound like? A series of scary drop pieces falling into place? The commercials on the easy listening radio station played in the reception room? The song by the Fifth Dimension your patients painfully associate with breaking up with their high school sweetheart playing on the "oldies" radio station? The less-then-forthcoming patient conversations heard through the hollow-core adjusting room doors? The lack of privacy when discussing financial matters at the front desk? The loud IBM Selectric typewriter inches away from the headache patients in the reception room?

Everything in a chiropractic office should contribute to its purpose.

Leave nothing to chance. Every sensory input, whether sight, sound, taste, touch, or smell should add to the patient's understanding of chiropractic and reveal or contribute to your purpose. Make sure new patients get the message that not only are they likely to get the pain relief they seek, but many patients remain under care and adopt a "chiropractic lifestyle." What senses are you engaging to send this message powerfully and congruently to patients in your office?

In the visual domain, the first picture affecting a patient's compliance is the exterior appearance of your office. What signal does it send to patients? Does the clinic sign feature the word "chiropractor" as if chiropractic was a consistently uniform commodity like pork bellies and sugar, or is the doctor's name more prominent?

What's the first impression new patients get when they walk through the front door? What year is it in your office? Do the colors and furnishings suggest a 1970s out-of-touch-earth-tone-beige or a "we're-in-touch-with-reality" contemporary color scheme? Are the magazines current, organized, and in good condition? Does it feel comfortable, safe, and human? Is the business office behind the front desk organized and efficient or in disorder? In mere seconds a new patient sizes up the doctor's attitude, attention to detail, and credibility with a single glance from the front door.

Are the brochures in your reception room full of pictures or a sea of type? Most chiropractic brochures work so hard at getting the chiropractic dogma correct, that little energy is given to the visuals that accompany the words. Instead, patients see the 1960s clip art illustration or 1970s black and white photography on the cover and decide they'd rather not spend the considerable effort to plow through the copy. No wonder your patients prefer *People* magazine!

The real opportunity to use specifically chosen visuals to communicate chiropractic occurs during the patient's report of findings. Are you using pictures of cracks in a foundation, orthodontic braces, the Tin Man from the *Wizard of Oz*, or a front end alignment to a car to explain spinal kinesiopathology? Are you using artifacts like a phone cable or the smell from a burnt electrical wire to communicate nervous system damage? Have you put your dimmer switch in your report of findings room yet? Have you picked up a rock with barnacles on it from your last trip to the beach to better explain the remodeling of bone spurs? The list is endless. Harness your creativity and make your chiropractic message more visual.

We learn about the world through our five senses. Offices that use as many senses as possible in their patient communications have more fun and their patients are more likely to understand and remember the chiropractic message. As long as you are held hostage by what patients might think about scented headrest paper, your antique rusty hinge used to demonstrate spinal degeneration, or your other innovative tools, you shortchange the impact your communications can have. Moreover, you compromise your role as a teacher — the true meaning of the word doctor. ■

MASLOW'S
CHIROPRACTIC

Are you one of those chiropractic doctors who recognize the value of a chiropractic lifestyle and encourage patients to remain under some type of on-going maintenance or wellness care? Often it seems like an uphill battle. Many patients seem to prefer pain relief over optimal health. Patients respond to the opportunity of maintenance care based on many factors not readily apparent to doctors. These factors include waiting time, cost of care, location, convenience, and dozens of other aspects of personality, bedside manner, and office procedures. If identified, many of these "interferences" to the accessibility and attractiveness of maintenance chiropractic care can be removed or avoided. But there's something much more pervasive that's standing in your way; Maslow and the hierachy of needs.

Remove the trappings of today's busy lifestyle and culture and look at the basics. At the most fundamental level we are motivated by the access to food and water. If these rudimentary supplies are available in a quantity and quality that assure our continued survival, then and only then are we motivated to pursue the next higher level of needs.

Clothing, followed by shelter, followed by security push further upward on Maslow's chart. Just about every patient who makes it into your office has these basics under control. The type and quality of clothing vary from patient to patient, as does their home—some rent some own. But what about security?

What if a patient loses his or her job or goes through a security-wrenching divorce? Are they likely candidates for non-symptomatic wellness chiropractic care? Probably not. Their security needs take precedence. This is why patients, especially blue collar patients who "make their living with their backs," can be quite motivated to follow through during the relief stages of care when their livelihood and mortgage payments are in jeopardy due to an incident or accident! For many of these patients, continuing their chiropractic care beyond the initial pain relief stage doesn't directly advance or contribute to the achievement of their security. Many of these patients rarely feel secure enough to rise any higher on Maslow's hierarchy of needs, continuing to exist month to month, paycheck to paycheck.

Progressing higher up the chart after security, Maslow placed the concept of companionship. Above that, the nurturing of one's self-esteem. Rarely does chiropractic contribute to one's self-esteem sufficiently enough to be a motivator. More about that later.

At the very top of the list, Maslow placed "self-actualization" or "self-improvement." Certainly chiropractic can help bring out all of one's potential. That's a natural reaction to having an optimally functioning nervous system.

Maslow suggests that one doesn't progress to the next higher "level" until needs are met at their current level. In other words, you aren't motivated to develop your self-esteem until the basics of food, shelter, and security are taken care of. What does this mean for chiropractors interested in developing a wellness practice of non-symptomatic patients/clients interested in optimizing their lives?

Let's face it. Patients who respect themselves, are inner directed, and want the best for themselves are fun patients to be around. They rarely whine about their sleepless nights or problems paying your bill because their rent is due. When patients hit the higher plains of esteem and actualization they are often more financially secure and pleasant to be around.

The challenge is to help move a patient from pain relief (security) to wellness (self-actualization). It's a big jump. And virtually impossible for doctors to make if they haven't reached the self-actualization stage themselves! That's a key point. Doctors who still have sweaty palms over making payroll or paying their malpractice insurance premiums will find it difficult to establish the necessary rapport to encourage their patients to enjoy the self-actualization that wellness care can promise.

According to Maslow, the step above security is companionship. Instead of a mating relationship, in the context of chiropractic it refers to the doctor/patient relationship. The doctor's bedside manner and ability to establish rapport without judgment are critical. This seems easier for doctors who can concentrate on truly serving their patients rather than seeing them as a $35 adjustment plus $30 for two therapies. On the other hand, doctors who lack an outgoing personality or who secretly resent the control their patients exert over their own security can never help their patients transcend this "companionship" level.

Improving one's self-esteem is the next higher level. Again, this is difficult for a doctor to develop in patients if he or she lack a high self worth themselves! If doctors are being held back at the companionship level because they want their patients to "like" them, it's difficult to mentor their patients' self-esteem. That's what's so powerful by unconditionally giving in the service of others. It liberates us to see others more clearly. We don't have the inclination to build a public relations campaign, worrying about what they'll think—we simply give. This unconditional attitude of service is powerful evidence to patients that you value them; maybe more than they value themselves. This is the prerequisite of facilitating the patients' self-esteem.

There are many opportunities to help improve a patient's self-esteem in a chiropractic setting. Besides the obvious wisdom of not condemning a patient for missing an appointment, forgetting their exercises, or parking in the wrong place, start using more praise. Make it a habit to compliment every patient on every visit, even if it's just the colors they wear or the fact they were on time. As an exclamation after their adjustment say, "You did great!" or some other form of congratulations. When you're running late, apologize, making them feel their time is more valuable than yours. The key is to respect each patient more perhaps than they respect themselves—while remaining genuine and sincere.

Another consideration is that patients who have a high level of self-esteem have higher expectations of you and your office, regardless of their symptomatic picture. These patients refuse to be treated like a number or to frequent an office with the ambiance of a bus station. The doctor and staff must have high self-esteem and project it in every thing they do, from the types of magazines chosen for the reception room and the type of language used by the staff, to the subtle qualities expressed in telephone manners and millions of little details about the office.

One must first have a relatively high level of self-esteem (a rare phenomenon these days) to be a candidate for the self-actualization represented by the desire to enjoy wellness chiropractic care. The self-actualization required to fulfill one's potential is a tall order for someone still worried about making the car payment and clothing their children. Most doctors are beyond these basic survival needs and can afford to "work on themselves" by optimizing their diets, exercise, and spinal biomechanics. If you have a hard time understanding why patients don't follow through with maintenance care, try to remember back what it was like to take a full course load as a student, hold a part time job, and share the rent with three friends. When one's security is threatened or unstable, it's difficult to selfishly squander one's resources on lofty intangibles such as personal development or self-actualization.

If you want more wellness patients you have to help grow them or begin a concerted marketing effort to attract patients who have high self-esteem and are ready for self-actualization opportunities. There must be a demand for quality chiropractic care among artists, thinkers, and gold collar workers in your community. But perhaps a better strategy would be to help grow more of these ideal patients by helping them reach higher levels of self-development while they are within your sphere of influence. When you help your patients think more highly of themselves and show them the possibilities for them and their families, you change the patient in a most positive way. It doesn't happen overnight. However, the trust and confidence they place in you because of the power of chiropractic offers a tremendous opportunity to change the world. ■

RAPPORT + RESULTS + RETENTION = REFERRALS

Regardless of technique, political persuasion, length of time in practice, or geographical location, the one thing that most doctors share in common is the desire for more new patients. How to get them eludes many doctors, especially those who still cling to the practice-building techniques that worked when insurance was plentiful and deductibles were low. Getting more new patients today requires new approaches. It's not business as usual.

First, recognize that having lots of new patients is a symptom. And not having lots of new patients is a symptom. Treating a lack of new patients medically, by treating its symptoms, would lead a doctor to squander time, money, and energy on everything from larger yellow page ads, mall shows, and free spinal exams to direct mail, giveaways, and bent pens! These approaches may generate people with spines, but they rarely attract the types of patients most doctors would like to grow their practices with.

Secondly, until you know why patients get great results in your office but don't refer others, your attempts to grow your practice will be a guess or a gimmick. Short term solutions that fail to address the underlying causes of a lack of new patients are destined to fail. Your patients know why they don't refer others. Until *you* know why and are willing to face the music, you're likely to continue sabotaging the natural referral process that produces the best kinds of patients.

When patients enter your practice, get great results, and drop out they are "firing" you. Unfortunately, you don't get a pink slip with an explanation so you can take corrective action. Today's patients vote with their feet. They don't owe you an explanation. They will rarely pull you aside during the rush hour to critique your report of findings or offer suggestions for eliminating capacity blockages. Don't confuse their nonverbal feedback as a lack of awareness! Patients are much more sensitive to how your office runs than you think. "He's a great doctor, but..." "She's a wonderful doctor, but..." That's what the referral dialogue in many offices sounds like. Are you willing to uncover and confront your patients' perceptions about you, your office, your procedures, your staff, your bedside manner, and millions of other "moments of truth" about your practice? Unless you're willing to get real, effortless practice growth will elude you.

A vital practice full of patients is the result of handling millions of details properly. Few of these essential details are taught in chiropractic colleges. It is a testimony to the power of chiropractic that thousands of practitioners have successful practices without learning the basics of successful practice in school! Instead of reading, 'riting, and 'rithmetic, the three Rs in chiropractic include rapport, results, and retention. It's the only formula that will generate the referrals licensed professionals seek.

Rapport: Rapport means more than just patient education and a meeting of the minds. It starts with personality. Do you have one? Frame all 21 diplomas and awards and hang them on your exam room wall and if you lack a personality, patients still don't connect with the office. While patients find it reassuring that the doctor graduated from these various institutions, what patients really care about is the reassurance, respect, and bedside manner that communicate hope and understanding.

An open communication style can even overcome sloppy clinical skills. How else can you explain classmates who barely passed the boards who have hugely successful offices? Until there is a course at chiropractic colleges entitled Tableside Manners 101, poor communications will sabotage some of the best chiropractic clinicians.

Results: It goes without saying that if you want an ample supply of new patients you must get consistent results with the patients that show up in your office. If you don't meet the expectations (pain relief) of your current patients, don't expect them to refer others. But it takes more than great results to have a successful practice. After almost 100 years of chiropractic history, it's clear that if all it took was great results, chiropractic would be at the top of the health care heap.

Patients don't really have results until they understand what's happened to them. Otherwise, their lack of involvement won't precipitate the passion and enthusiasm necessary to prompt them to refer others. In fact, you must exceed their expectations (pain relief) to generate the top-of-mind-awareness necessary for patients to tell others about chiropractic with evangelical fervor. And while it's true that many of your "miracle" cases seem powerless to coax others to your office, at the root of their problem is often a lack of patient education. *If your patients can't explain chiropractic, overcome the common myths and misconceptions about chiropractic, and defend their chiropractic decision, it's unlikely they'll reveal their chiropractic identity to others.* This is pretty basic stuff. But ask most chiropractors what they do—and they can't tell you. "I align the spine." "I remove subluxations." "I adjust the spine." "I help restore a patient's natural inborn healing ability."

Huh?

Until chiropractors *and* their patients can adequately explain chiropractic without depending upon jargon, chiropractic will remain a second class, alternative, natural-form-of-pain-relief profession. Symptomatic improvement produces happy patients, but only patient education empowers patients to confidently refer others.

Retention: How long do patients remain under care in your office? How many understand chiropractic well enough to become chiropractic clients? Client relationships are much more enjoyable and create the environment that can better nurture the referral process.

A pain-relief outlook is generally short term. Medicine has taught patients that the objective of health care is to avoid pain or discomfort. If patients enter your practice with this myopic vision of health, your patient education efforts should be designed to reveal the benefits of a chiropractic lifestyle. Worse, is when chiropractors adopt this limited view and think they are doing patients a favor by quickly getting them symptom free and dismissing them. Without proper education to change their expectations, the reemergence of their symptoms from their under-lying chronic condition months or years later, leaves patients with the notion that chiropractic doesn't work or is merely an expensive short-term fix.

Don't misunderstand. If, after exposing patients to a wellness ap-proach to health it is rejected, honor them, willingly dismiss them, and thank them for the opportunity to participate with them in their symptomatic recovery. The crime is in not exposing patients to the benefits of the same chiropractic lifestyle you enjoy!

Long-term doctor/patient/client relationships are only possible when affordable wellness care fees are available and your procedures are efficient so as not to excise large amounts of time. Patients are not living to get adjusted! Patients get adjusted so they can go live.

When patients refer their friends they're putting their friendships on the line for you. When they vouch for you, they are staking their reputation for yours. From the first impression of walking into your reception area, to the last ditch reactivation efforts by your well-inten-tioned staff, your patients are sizing you up. The conclusions they reach will not only direct their own compliance, but will hinder or advance their willingness to tell others about their experience in your office. Perhaps more sobering, these conclusions will affect their perception of the entire chiropractic profession. Is it possible that today you're paying the price of the new patient gimmicks used in the past? What legacy are you leaving the next generation of chiropractors and chiropractic patients? ■

ADJUSTMENT ETIQUETTE

There is a generally accepted mode of behavior that governs our interactions with each other. These social skills or "rules" can be defined by situation, environment, age, even the time of day. Often this code of conduct remains unspoken, isolating newcomers and making beginners uncomfortable. In fact, these rules can intimidate those with low self-esteem and prevent many from trying new experiences. Encountering three forks at a restaurant, attending a black tie affair, or ordering Chinese food are common examples. The newcomer or neophyte must be extremely sensitive to read the clues to fit in.

When we are in a new and uncomfortable situation, we are always grateful to those who will take us under their wing and show us the ropes. This guide and mentor paves the way for us to enjoy the situation and fit in easier. For a new patient, fitting in and getting acclimated to chiropractic can be intimidating. Just what are your expectations of patients in the adjustment room, and what do you suppose their expectations are of you? Do you explain your adjustment room etiquette to your patients—in advance?

Because patients can't consult a book entitled something like, *Emily Post for the Adjusting Room*, here are some issues you might want to take into consideration with your next new patient.

First visit expectations: Create a simple outline of the major events of a patient's first visit experience. List the typical office procedures, explaining why they are performed and the benefits to the patient. Patient rapport is improved and you'll discover patients become more cooperative. Volunteering this information in a consistent manner will make patients more receptive and in the end, more appreciative of your thoughtfulness.

Adjusting room greeting: How do you greet patients on routine visits? "How are you doing?" "How's your health?" Regardless of how you ask it, what type of response do you really want from the patient? Do you want a listing of purely physical complaints, raves about how wonderful the last adjustment was or wasn't, or a recitation that includes car troubles and a weather forecast? Your expectations create the tone of your relationship with the patient. Will you be living and breathing chiropractic on every visit? Do you have other interests? Are you insecure about the progress of the relationship? Explain to patients in advance what type of information, and why, you'll want to know on each visit.

Examination findings: It surprises me how many doctors who do leg length checks, motion palpation, and other tests on every visit consistently fail to tell the patient what they're discovering. Whether doctors think patients don't care, wouldn't understand, or just hadn't thought about it, is hard to say. The more you involve the patient, the more you improve compliance and follow through. Help patients know what you know!

Can we talk? Does one talk before, during, or after the adjustment? Does the doctor need to concentrate—so please no interruptions? Will you be asking questions you want answered while the patient's jaw is wedged between the headrest paper? Let patients know how you prefer to handle conversation during the adjusting process.

Eyes open or closed? Does this matter? Is there anything you want patients to be thinking about or visualizing during the adjustment? Give patients some guidance, or if it doesn't matter, at least talk about it. Patients wonder, even though they might not ask about it.

I give you a "9.5." Does the doctor want a critique of the adjustment after it is delivered? Do we talk about it? Does the doctor care? This issue may reveal more about the doctor's self-confidence than any other. Do you want this valuable feedback loop, or, do you not care what patients think about your adjusting style? While you probably don't want patients holding up numbered cards like Olympic freestyle diving judges use, some type of feedback is valuable. Patients know what they want, especially if they've been to other chiropractors.

Right side/left side: "Now, I'd like you to turn with your left side up." That's not how our brains work when lying horizontal on your table. How about touching the side you want up? We're generally in a kinesthetic mode while receiving our adjustments and touching would be a big help.

Privacy: Many patients in focus groups mention this aspect. Patients want privacy. That may simply mean having a professional carpenter replace your hollow core door with the 2" gap at the bottom with a solid core door that fits. In open office environments it may mean investing in a pink or white noise generator to mask conversations or reminding patients of your private office for more sensitive conversations. Without privacy the doctor/patient relationship is compromised and is no deeper than that we have with our barber.

Buying time or talent? Are patients made to believe they are buying a certain amount of time and attention from the doctor? "My last chiropractor spent 15 minutes with me for $30," said one patient in a recent focus group. Are you selling time, which is easy to do, especially when starting in practice when you do have so much time? If you do, it's a dangerous trap if you want to be a major influence in your community. Let patients know that because of your experience with hundreds, perhaps thousands of patients, you will only need about X minutes to correct their spinal biomechanics. Since their time is valuable, you're going to help them as quickly as you can, so they can get on with their lives.

These are just a few of the issues that surround an even broader and more interesting concept I call a doctor's adjusting room "tableside manners." It's based on the doctor's social skills, personality, technique, communication skills, sense of time, appearance, and many other characteristics. Adjusting room etiquette and these other issues profoundly affect the patients' trust in you, their willingness to comply with your recommendations, and ultimately, their desire to refer others to your office. ∎

THE PERCEPTION OF TIME

One of the reasons why patients don't opt for continued maintenance care is because the care you provide takes too long to get. Many offices function under the misguided notion that patients are most concerned about the length of time they spend in the reception room. And while this aspect is important, it is like the seven blind men feeling different parts of the elephant and perceiving an elephant to be different than it really is. How patients perceive the time spent in your office changes during the course of their care.

First Appointment Time

Because of a lack of understanding about chiropractic, or apprehensions about consulting a "bad back" doctor, many patients neglect their spines or wait until they are desperate before making the first phone call to your office. some new patients wait until their fear of the stroke or paralysis they've heard chiropractic care could cause, is eclipsed by their discomfort. Finally, they have nothing to lose! As the insurance industry continues to crumble and the economy remains tight, you'll notice this problem will get worse. Consider the challenges of building rapport with an increasing number of patients who are incapacitated and in a hurry for relief so the financial burden of care can be lifted!

This, combined with the "one-visit-for-the-high-powered-prescription" belief they've been taught by their medical doctor, sets the stage for an uncomfortable first-visit scrimmage played out in many offices.

The unfortunate results of these misunderstandings endanger compliance, retention, referrals, and the healing process.

For new patients, time is measured by how long it takes for pain relief. During this earliest stage of care go easy on the chiropractic science and philosophy. Communicate hope while explaining the reasonable expectations they should have, based on similar cases in your office. Ask patients for a length of time that they'd be willing to suspend judgment to allow chiropractic care to work. Will they give it five visits? Fifteen visits? Get a large enough commitment so there's a good chance they'll sense some progress, but small enough that you don't confirm their fear that "once you start you have to go for the rest of your life." Use those initial visits to educate the patient and enlarge their understanding and appreciation of a chiropractic lifestyle.

Routine Visit Time

As their symptomatic picture improves and their visits become more routine, the patient's perception of time changes again. Now comfortable with you, your staff, and your office procedures, coming to the office has become a pleasant diversion for the day. The urgency of the earlier visits has been replaced with a more relaxed mood. Many patients spend more time socializing during this period of their care and devour your reception room magazines. Some are even put out when they are called to an adjusting room in the middle of an article about some prominent celebrity's latest heartbreak. Time in your office is a refuge from the real world. Where else can you go these days and have your insurance pay for being loved, cared for, and really appreciated?

Of course if you're paying out of your own pocket for these visits, the perceptions are much different! Without effective patient education and streamlined office procedures, this is when many cash-paying patients jump ship. What started out as an effective form of natural pain relief has turned into an expensive and indulgent personal luxury. It's not the time they're wasting by being in your office in a relatively non-symptomatic state, it's a financial consideration. If patients send you signals that suggest they don't feel worthy of continued non-symptomatic care, it may be time to consider using the Häagen-Dazs Strategy.

In Faith Popcorn's book, *The Popcorn Report*, she describes a trend called "Small Indulgences." It's based on the notion that while most of us eat ice cream, more and more we're doing it as a reward for being good. We tell ourselves we've been good little boys or girls and we reward ourselves with a more expensive premium brand. It's a small indulgence we've earned by being so good the other six days of the week.

When patients are feeling better and finances cloud the issue of rehabilitative or wellness care, it may be wise to adapt this approach to their continued chiropractic care. "I'm delighted you're feeling better Bob, and while we haven't been able to work on repatterning and reeducating the associated soft tissue involvement, we'll always be here. Stop by once a month or so and allow us to pamper you with some type of continued chiropractic care so you're less likely to suffer a relapse."

Maintenance Care Time

Now both time and money issues change again. Most offices with lots of cash-paying wellness patients have developed some type of wellness care fee arrangement in their office. If you want more of these types of patients, you must give some thought to how you're going to make non-symptomatic preventive care affordable. Your usual and customary adjusting fee is too expensive for someone who is feeling fine.

If getting wellness care adjustments exact too high a price in terms of the amount of time in your office, maintenance patients will be less inclined to return several times a month for a tune-up. Using the old yardstick of measuring reception room waiting time is no longer effective. Instead, measure Door Slam Time.

Door Slam Time is the elapsed time from when patients slam their car door to step into your office, to the time they slam their car door to get on with their life. Forget about the Disney notion of "keeping the line moving" or "storing patients" in drab adjusting rooms with double digit plastic numbers glued on the doors! What patients are measuring is how much total time out of their increasingly busy lives does it take to get adjusted? How much time are patients spending when they slam their car doors at 5:15 P.M. and march into your office? Put a watch to it. Is the cost of maintenance care in your office, in terms of either time or money, preventing patients from adopting a chiropractic lifestyle?

If you want to help manage your patients' perceptions of time and so you can better meet or exceed their expectations, it first takes a sensitivity to a patient's concept of time, and the willingness to consistently communicate these issues. Here are two suggestions:

1. "Why did you wait 34 years before coming in?" Many of the underlying causes of spinal-related health problems in adults got started at birth or in childhood. "Ever fall off a bicycle or out of a tree?" Explain the adaptive qualities of the body and how their current symptomatology may be the result of some uncorrected event that occurred years ago. Help patients put their current health complaint into a longer-term perspective, rather than "something happened when I bent over last week."

2. "How long do you think it took for that bone spur to form?" Again, this helps reposition their expectations for recovery since their problem has obviously existed for longer than the last couple of months they've been getting headaches. An effective approach many dentists use is to compare the "age" of the patient's teeth and gums with the patient's chronological age. "Mrs. Smith, you have a pretty good spine for a 65 year-old, but it says here that you'll be 42 in September!" Buy time for your chiropractic care recommendations to work by explaining the consequences of their previous neglect. After all, it's their spinal problem, not yours.

While you can never be sure if these metaphors can help change a patient's perception of time, there are things you can do to help reduce office time as an issue affecting patient compliance throughout the stages of their care:

1. Measurement: Increase your awareness of time-related issues by having your staff record each patient's reception room waiting time and door slam time. In small print in the appointment book record the time each patient walks in the front door (W1), the time they "go to the back room" (W2), and the time they walk out the front door (W3). Then plot the elapsed Reception Room Waiting Time (W2-W1) and the total elapsed Door Slam Time (W3-W1) throughout the day. (You may need to instruct your staff to do these measurements secretly so you don't change your behavior and corrupt their findings.) Get reliable information to motivate you to implement some of the following suggestions and then remeasure several months later.

2. Sell your talent not time. How long does it take to adjust your spouse? Why do you spend so much longer adjusting your patients? Make sure patients understand they're buying your talent, not your time! "Because I've been at this for 12 years, Mrs. Jones, and I have delivered hundreds of thousands of adjustments, it's going to take me about three and a half minutes to evaluate your condition and adjust you on your future visits. Now, I can stretch it out to 10 or 12 minutes, but if I do, I can't help as many people as I'd like to and you've probably got better things to do than to talk about the weather, or who won the game last night. So with your permission, I'd prefer to give you 100% of my focused attention and experience so you can go enjoy your new health. Now, at any time you'd like to discuss any aspect of your health or treatment in our office, I'd be honored to invest the time to answer any questions." If you'll just explain why and remind them of the benefits of brief visits, most new patients will be delighted.

3. Compute the value of a minute. This is an eye-opener for doctors who squander valuable time because they're unaware of it's real cost (or worth). How much is your time worth when you're in high gear at 5:30 P.M.? Not that money should be the basis of every office decision, however, remind yourself of this figure the next time you're talking about the weather or sports scores with a patient. Take the total collections during the peak hour of your day and divide by sixty.

4. Reduce physical barriers. Now that you know how much a minute costs, how much does it cost you to take the ten steps from adjusting room one to adjusting room three? How much does it cost to open and close a needless door? How much does that eight second ride up and the eight second ride down on your adjusting table take? Am I being too petty? You decide. But when I ask patients in focus groups how "full" they perceive the office to be at the time they get adjusted and I hear 90% or 95% full, the choice is to work at removing capacity blockages that are measured in seconds, hire the management headaches of an associate, work on growing the off-peak hours, or resign yourself to the fact that your office is as big as it's ever going to get.

In the old days when everyone had $100 deductibles and didn't stay for preventive care, it was easy to run the office because for the most part all the patients had similar perceptions of time. A fifteen minute wait in the reception room, a seven minute encounter with the doctor, some unsupervised therapy and presto, they were on their way. Today, as deductibles soar and fewer patients even have insurance, adapting your office procedures and wisely spending your patient's time resources are more essential than ever. ∎

SEVEN REASONS PATIENTS DON'T REFER

When you got involved in chiropractic, you implicitly or explicitly accepted the notion of looking for cause rather than treating symptoms. Regardless of which chiropractic college you attended, you were introduced to a perspective so radical, yet so simple that you probably take it for granted now. The role of the nervous system in controlling health (function) is a new idea for most patients.

Getting to cause instead of treating symptoms is a perspective helpful in virtually any endeavor. Yet, we are a culture of symptom treaters. All too many parents treat the symptoms of their children's poor behavior instead of the cause. Instead of ferreting out the cause of frequent speeding tickets we treat the symptom with a radar detector. Rather than confront the cause of being overweight we buy something, join an organization, or distract ourselves in some other way. Denial becomes so ingrained in our behavior that real solutions to our problems are obscured. Our behavior becomes a series of rationalizations that make us feel trapped and alone.

It's interesting that a profession that ascribes to finding the cause of a patient's health care problem and avoids treating the symptom, is rift with doctors treating the symptoms of a less than optimum practice! Poor compliance is a symptom. High staff turnover is a symptom. Low patient volume is a symptom. However, the solutions prescribed by management specialists or the "I-had-a-great-practice-once" seminar lecturers rarely offer approaches that attack the true cause of these common frustrations.

We pay dearly when we are lied to. First we pay to attend seminars so someone can whisper sweet nothings into our ears. Then we pay again when their advice backfires or is so personality dependent as to be non-information.

We are constantly on the lookout so we can blame causes outside our own responsibility. The snowstorm. The economy. The small rural community. The A.M.A. The insurance companies. The paperwork. The HMOs and PPOs. The chiropractor down the street. Yellow page ad placement. Being the youngest child. Being the oldest child. Being too short. Not having enough time.

Have I missed any?

When patients look outside for solutions (drugs and surgery) and when doctors look outside (excuses and rationalizations) they rarely get lasting results.

If growing a practice, like healing, is an inside job, it's necessary to look inside the practice for the cause(s) thwarting the natural referral process. That means looking at the doctor, the patients, the staff, and the physical surroundings of the office itself. Here are some common, yet often overlooked causes for a lack of referrals:

1. Poor doctor/patient rapport: Improving a patient's spinal bio-mechanics is more than just a clinical procedure. The doctor's personality and communication skills play a larger role than most doctors think. Doctors must walk the fine line between being a "friend" and being a clinician. This balance is difficult for the analytical and the technique guru who measure success with a protractor. Don't expect a lot of referrals if patients perceive you as distant, preoccupied, or unenthusiastic. Make sure your passion about chiropractic and your hope for the patient is continually obvious.

2. Patients lack the words to refer: Can you describe chiropractic without using the words "subluxation," "adjustment," "fixation," and other language that most prospective chiropractic patients have never heard before? One of the easiest detectable reasons why patients don't refer is because they don't have a way to describe what goes on in your office to others. That's why some form of systematic, relentless patient education is so critical. If patients can only describe their chiropractic experience by how they "feel," they will be severely limited in their ability to tell others what chiropractic is and be confident fielding the inevitable questions.

3. Can't defend their decision: More subtle is the peer pressure that prevents many chiropractic patients from telling others. The alternative-not-approved-last-resort-cultist-charismatic image that chiropractic suffers from, stops many image-conscious chiropractic patients from revealing their chiropractic identity to others. Even patients who get phenomenal results are often closed-mouthed about chiropractic. It's not cool enough. It suggests poor judgment if one has been swayed by some non-mainstream practitioner who offers free exams and uses coupons to solicit new patients. Because few patients are equipped to explain why chiropractors are seemingly not allowed to prescribe drugs, or detail a chiropractor's educational achievements, or counter the dozen other myths and misconceptions about the profession, they don't say a word. It's easier that way.

4. Nothing worth talking about: When you do something (or don't do something) that doesn't meet a patient's expectations it causes negative word of mouth about your practice. "He/She's a great doctor but..." When you exceed a patient's expectations it causes positive word of mouth. "You gotta come meet my chiropractor because..." When you simply meet a patient's expectations there is no word of mouth. In all too many offices this is a major obstacle to more referrals. There's nothing extraordinary to talk about. If you want your patients to be compelled to tell others you must romance your office, your procedures, and every aspect of a patient's encounter with chiropractic so it exceeds a patient's expectations. Start by holding a staff meeting devoted to making a list of the expectations of today's quality- and time-conscious new patient. Then brainstorm ways of exceeding those expectations in a consistent and systematic way.

5. Lack of patient education: Many chiropractic patients think chiropractic is appropriate only for the complaint for which they consulted your office. No wonder low back patients refer other low back cases and headache patients only refer headache patients. And why so few children receive care in chiropractic offices. Besides the short-term goal of improving compliance and speeding the healing process, patient education should broaden a patient's understanding of chiropractic so they see its almost universal appropriateness. Without patient education, conventional wisdom would suggest most children don't need chiropractic care. Without patient education, your patients can't explain chiropractic or answer a friend's well-intentioned questions.

6. Referral efforts aren't rewarded: Human Nature 101 suggests that what gets done is what gets rewarded. Want more referrals? Reward this positive behavior in a way that gets a patient's attention! The Thank-You Gram, name on the referral board, and free adjustment aren't as dramatic and as appreciated today as they once were. Funny how many offices that still use these uncreative techniques are the same ones squandering thousands of dollars on advertising! If you've ever watched a patient count the number of names on your sign in sheet and multiply it by the cost of care, you know that they know what a new patient is worth. Up the ante and say thank you in a more memorable way. Consider a tickets to movies, sporting events, concerts and other cultural activities. Perhaps certificates for car washes, a massage, having one's "colors done," or some other indulgence. Other patients might enjoy an evening in a limousine, a harbor cruise, singing telegram, or a champagne breakfast hot air balloon ride. Use your creativity to say "thank you" in a creative and memorable way.

7. Office capacity already reached: Most of us are quite selfish. Why introduce others to chiropractic so we have to wait even longer for our care? Every factory, business, or service provider has some type of capacity limitations. It may be legal, physical, psychological, procedural, or some other restriction. Patients are more sensitive to the capacity of your office than you think. Ask patients "how full" they perceive your office to be at the time they receive their care. The higher the percentage, the more unlikely patients will refer others. If the limitations you've assumed or imposed on your practice cannot be changed, start working on strategies to increase your off-peak practice hours.

There are some in chiropractic who make the point that if you want more referrals, you need to ask patients for them. That's treating a potential symptom. Consultants who recommend heavy-handed approaches and super-duper-this-will-get-patients-to-refer scripts often accuse reluctant doctors of an "unwillingness to confront" if they don't panhandle their current patients for referrals. There is a reason why patients don't refer. Simply asking them doesn't get to the cause. In fact, it puts patients in an uncomfortable position. They resent divulging the name of a close friend or business associate, not only because of one or more of the reasons mentioned earlier, but because they can reasonably expect you'll treat their friends in the same heavy-handed way you're treating them!

Reminding patients of their responsibility to tell others about chiropractic needn't be uncomfortable or manipulative. "I'm so glad you're doing better Mrs. Jones. Now, because you know more about chiropractic than probably any of your friends, be sure to let them know how we can help." Most patients would find a low key approach such as this to be perfectly professional and warranted.

Want more love? Don't whine to others that no one loves you. Become a better lover yourself. Want more new patients? You don't ask. Become worthy of the risk patients take when they vouch for you by telling their friends. Until you see your practice through the eyes of your patients, the lack of referrals will remain a better kept secret than chiropractic itself! ■

BEYOND THE BOX
ON THE WALL

Even doctors who stress patient education, do regular patient lectures, and consider themselves excellent communicators find that patients drop out of care. The fact that this "premature dismissal" generally coincides with the patient reaching symptomatic improvement can lead many doctors to think that rehabilitative and wellness care is something no one wants. But that would over simplify and ignore a very important issue that becomes more obvious when you see your practice through the eyes of a typical patient.

In the "old days" before insurance equality, but after the donation box-on-the-wall method of chiropractic compensation, there was generally one fee for an adjustment. Didn't matter if it was the patient's first adjustment or the hundredth. The fee was the fee and it was largely determined by what the market would bear and influenced by the local cost of living. If you practiced in Westchester County, New York you generally charged more for an adjustment than if you practiced in Billings, Montana.

It was a good time for chiropractic because there was focus. Doctors were not distracted by narratives that go unread, the expense and overhead caused by computers, nor were they combating the latest foot-dragging tactics of the insurance companies. The staff was few in number and didn't require seminars, bonuses, and incentives to fuel their commitment. It was a simpler time and the emphasis was on the chiropractic adjustment and personal service. Chiropractic was more likely to be a family affair for most patients. Entire families would file into the adjusting room to receive their care. It was a time of huge practices. Some chiropractors even had private airstrips to accommodate patients that would fly in from around the world. Chiropractors who had gone to jail for practicing their healing art were still fresh in everyone's memory.

Today, the vision of many chiropractic doctors is so limited they don't even bother printing their telephone area code on their business cards or letterhead!

Some would claim that insurance equality laws opened the doors of chiropractic to patients who would have never tried it. Others suggest that the insurance industry "legitimized" chiropractic. Both are probably correct to some degree. Yet this same industry is a contributing factor in the prevailing sickness orientation seen in most chiropractic offices, and the decrease in the number of families, children, and maintenance patients receiving care today. If chiropractic gets limited to the twelve visit-symptomatic-relief-only box suggested by the RAND Study and a growing number of state legislatures are suggesting, it will be because of this all too willing alignment with the insurance industry.

As the number of patients with insurance dwindles and their deductibles rise, making a "chiropractic lifestyle" affordable for cash paying patients should be a prime concern of doctors interested in surviving and thriving in the years ahead. *Keeping* patients will become as important as getting new ones. Bragging rights at chiropractic get togethers won't be centered on new patient statistics, but retention and patient visit averages. For most offices, besides relentless patient education, it will require developing and implementing some type of wellness care fee system for people who want non-symptomatic maintenance care. Many patients drop out because they simply can't afford or justify paying your usual and customary sickness care fees when they're feeling fine. Until you make wellness (maintenance) care affordable, don't expect to enjoy the referrals, financial security, and satisfaction that comes from serving well patients who understand and respect what you do.

If chiropractic had never attained insurance "equality," there would be little need for a way to help make post symptomatic care affordable for people after they exhaust their insurance benefits.

All too many chiropractic doctors have become accustomed to $30, $40, or $50 adjustments. Still others add additional physical therapy charges (because insurance pays for it). Total visit charges in the $60-$90 range or higher are not unusual. X-rays with a 800% mark-up are common. And why not? The insurance company will pay it. When chiropractors allow themselves to be so strongly influenced by the "sickness care" mentality of insurance companies and start thinking anyone would gladly pay $30 for an adjustment, even when they feel fine, you have the crisis in chiropractic that we see today.

If all insurance coverage for chiropractic were eliminated tomorrow do you really think your fee structure would remain the same? Oh, maybe for a week or two, but in a "deregulated" practice environment more in touch with reality it wouldn't be business as usual. Doctors who are over-staffed or living a highly-leveraged lifestyle would like to believe otherwise. "I deserve it," they rationalize. "I endured four winters in Davenport," they moan. With the violins weeping, they set their fees to the upper reaches reported by *Fee Facts,* or what a quick phone survey of other doctors in their area uncovers. Then they greedily take whatever they can bill and collect for. Physical therapy? Does insurance pay for it? Let's do it. Rehab equipment? Does insurance pay for it? Let's get some. Mineral supplements? Does insurance pay for it? Let's add those too. Suddenly anything that fell under the state's scope of practice laws and was reimbursable by the patient's insurance policy became part of the patient's treatment plan. Interestingly, if the patient didn't have insurance or their policy limited these adjunctive procedures, they often weren't performed. The easiest way to predict a patient's care program would be to read the patient's insurance policy.

That's wrong.

Physical therapy isn't the issue. It's using a patient's financial resources as a guideline for making clinical recommendations. All the rationalizations in the world cannot cover up the fact that this is a form of stealing.

Is this why doctors these days have such a reluctance to look a patient in the eye and present their fees? Is this why staff members have such difficulty collecting money, unconsciously siding with patients because they know they couldn't afford to pay what they're being asked to collect?

The fact is chiropractors exist in an isolating subculture. Most enjoy a better standard of living than their patients. You've had a well-grounded education in physiology, so you understand the danger of aberrant spinal biomechanics. But perhaps more dangerous is the fact that you probably get your once a week or twice a month wellness adjustment without any impact to your monthly budget. Nor do you have to endure a crowded reception room at 5:30 to get it. This distorts your ability to see your practice the way cash-paying "well" patients see your practice.

You're too expensive.

This financial myopia has turned chiropractic into an expensive form of non-invasive pain relief. It's the last resort before back surgery. And increasingly the patient looks to their "you're-in-good-hands" insurance company for recommendations about appropriate chiropractic care.

If you want to divorce yourself from practicing medicine (treating symptoms and patients dismissing themselves), then develop ways patients can afford your care on a non-symptomatic basis. Create ways patients can afford wellness chiropractic care on the same visit frequency you do.

This generation of chiropractic patients, (and probably the next), bring a medical model of health with them to your office. Wellness care is a new idea for most. In fact, simply being healthy is a new idea! Because of this, most patients don't want to be truly healthy, they just want to live without pain or discomfort. That's why patient education is so important.

But incredible patient education isn't enough. Have you priced organically grown produce recently? Been shopping for meat and poultry raised without antibiotics and growth hormones? It's expensive to really care about your health. It's cheaper, easier, and faster to go to McDonald's. Cost creates a barrier that prevents patients who under-stand and want continued chiropractic care from getting it. Sure, patients should drive a less expensive car so they could afford to pay your fees. But they don't. And patients should be willing to delay gratification and be willing to pay for the often intangible and not immediately recognized benefits of wellness care. But they aren't.

Your response to what your patients *should* do versus what your patients actually do will determine the impact of your practice in years ahead. Perhaps it's time to take a more pragmatic view and question the status quo.

Of course patient education is paramount. Without patient education you could offer wellness care for free and still not have any takers. While we can cling to our philosophical "rightness" and expect insurance companies to pay for wellness care and desire true health for their customers, this is not the case. Yes, they will gladly pay thousands for ineffective back surgery, but not pay for the most minimal amounts of preventive care. Looking to an insurance company (a business—not a public utility) for any type of guidance is futile.

Hope springs eternal. If you're thinking some type of nationalized health care is going to be the solution, don't hold your breath. Remember, whatever emerges will be from the same folks who brought you Medicare!

Until chiropractic is better understood, utilized, and accepted by the general public, it will always be easy to cap it, limit it, or exclude it. Just ask doctors in Oregon, Colorado, Minnesota, and Canada. ■

STEP BY STEP DISENGAGEMENT

As you welcome your last $250 deductible insurance patient into your office and you hear the safety removed from the gun at your temple, celebrate what a wonderful decade it's been since insurance equality. Maybe take the office staff out for one last blow out, paid for by the $35 adjustments, $20 ice packs, and $275 Davis series. What's left of many offices resembles the morning after an all night party with the throbbing headache, dirty dishes, and the hollow emptiness the lingers after the last guest leaves. But the dry mouth and blurred vision isn't from enjoying yourself too much. For many, it's the primordial fight or flight kicking in: fear. Fear of the future.

If you've had enough of the paperwork, narratives, lost claims, delaying tactics, and minimum wage clerks passing judgment on your diagnosis and treatment plan, the choice is clear. Decide not to play the game. Decide to disengage from the insurance industry. It will cost you. But then freedom always exacts a price.

Who said you had to accept insurance assignment? Who says the patient expects it? Who says you need a computer? And the latest $3,500 software to run it? And the staff to feed it? And office space to house it? And the hassles? And the frustration of providing a wellness approach to health inside a sickness care model of insurance?

Try to remember how strange acquiring your insurance-related tools and office procedures felt years ago! It probably feels even more unsettling to entertain the thoughts of abandoning them now. Soon your computer will make an expensive door stop. Your therapy equipment? It probably won't be replaced when it breaks down or wears out. The thousands of square feet of office space? You could easily get by with less. You get the picture. Chiropractic will go through a simplification process. It will be cleansing and it will offer the bravest survivors a sense of freedom and fulfillment that 35 new patients a month with $100 deductibles could never match.

You've been practicing in a "regulated" environment. No one says you have to charge the same $30 usual and customary fee for an adjustment as every one else is, but with one eye on what the insurance companies will pay, it almost seems real. After all, "I'm worth it. I've paid my dues. And anyway, in the long run chiropractic care is less expensive than the back surgery insurance companies seem even more willing to pay for."

So as greed and pride cloud reason, we lose touch with reality. Detroit auto manufacturers who continue to overlook America's artificially low price of gasoline (Japanese drivers paid the equivalent of $3.25 a gallon in 1992), seem unmotivated to make cars with the fuel efficiency needed to face the future. This lack of awareness almost killed Chrysler, and none of the American manufacturers have a particularly healthy balance sheet. By the way, don't expect any loan guarantees or government bailouts for chiropractic!

I'm not a doomsdayer, but some drastic changes will be required of you and your practice. Those who cannot or will not adapt will be forced to leave the profession. Those who had marginal practices with the help of insurance will become "reborn", or become associates for more successful and adaptive doctors. And while many students will emerge from school with a huge debt service, they will not be burdened by expensive lifestyles or other insurance-fed habits. Because it will be easier, but more difficult at the same time, those who got into chiropractic for the wrong reasons, lack a strong chiropractic philosophy, or refuse to educate their patients, will probably be forced to get out of chiropractic. Similarities of this same shakeout process have already been seen in the computer, airline, and banking industries. The solvent companies swallow up the marginal, faltering smaller companies. The strong survive.

If it's not too late, here are some scenarios you may wish to consider as you consciously plan your escape from the influence of insurance. The common thread through all these approaches is the recognition that increasingly higher deductibles and the growing number of patients without insurance have removed chiropractic care from the reach of many patients who need and want it. Unless you want the stress and confusion that comes from creating a financial hardship arrangement with practically every new patient, it may be time to reorient your fees. Like making sausage, it's not pretty.

1. Financial hardship cases: As soon as virtually every cash patient is on a "hardship arrangement" it would be hard for a jury not to agree with the insurance companies that your hardship fee is your fee. Besides the confusion of tracking everyone's different fees, wait until Mrs. Smith finds out Mrs. Jones is paying less! Abuse this approach because it's expedient and prepare to refund already spent insurance checks!

2. You pay one, I'll pay one: As a few insurance cases linger, this strategy keeps your fees up while still allowing your cash patients to continue care. You simply "pay" for the visits they can't afford. If you thought keeping up with Medicare was fun, this ought to be right up your alley. While it might work in the short term, it's still treating a symptom: your fees are too high. Cash paying patients can't afford you.

3. Case management fees: This is where you offer cash patients a three or four month care program for their initial intensive and rehabilitative care that allows patients to budget equal monthly payments. This turnkey approach bundles any necessary examinations, X-rays, and adjustments into a single care package. During the first month or two visit frequency is high and the patient is ahead of you. During the last month or so they pay the same amount but their visit frequency is reduced, evening out the equation. Can you offer an arrangement like this without implying a cure?

4. Eliminate assignment: You could change this policy tomorrow. Let the patient extricate money from their insurance company. Some suggest helping the patient discover the cut off date on their credit cards and charging the card for their care, using the credit card "float" between billing cycles to buy time for the patient to receive the insurance check. I don't remember seeing Financial Manipulation 101 on the chiropractic college catalogs I've reviewed! Worse, wait for the first new patient to storm out of your office because the doctor down the street still takes assignment.

5. Miscellaneous: The jury is still out on some of the other schemes floating around the profession. I don't know if the "buy-eight-visits-get-ten" approach has been tested in court yet. The "bookkeeping discount" for cash paying patients attracts undue attention when it exceeds about 10% which is rarely enough of a price lowering to really help.

Before you jump out a window, relax knowing there is a solution. Cash. Greenbacks. Money. Bread. Dough. Moolah. That's right. The celebrated cash practice will finally arrive. The solution: one fee. Whether it's the patient's first adjustment or 122th adjustment. Whether they have insurance, HMO membership, or cash.

The only problem is your cash fee will probably be only two thirds or less of what your usual and customary charge is now.

Don't panic! And don't throw the baby out with the bath water. You'll know when it's time to deploy your parachute and go strictly to cash. Until then if I were in practice I'd take these preparatory steps:

A. Pay off as many debts as possible while adjusting your personal lifestyle.

B. Lower your overhead as much as possible without compromising patient care.

C. Attend seminars that stress chiropractic philosophy.

D. Commit yourself to optimum patient education.

E. Trust your judgment and avoid radical changes.

F. Visualize your practice full of cash paying patients.

Before the insurance company's final gasps you have the opportunity to adapt to this new practice environment and increase your chances of survival. And while it isn't fashionable to talk about "downward mobility" and "less is more," doctors with their eyes on the horizon and ears to the ground know big changes are coming. The question is, do you have the courage to take the necessary steps now to end your dependency on insurance and assume responsibility for the future? ■

TAKING RESPONSIBILITY

One day I discovered some strange stains on the walls of my four-year old's bedroom. "What happened?" I asked.

"I don't know," mumbled Eric evading my glance.

"What caused these funny stains on the wall?" I repeated.

There was a long pause. "The Ghostbusters were chasing a third class vapor and mutagen got stuck on the wall," he said with perfect diction and a completely serious expression.

I'd never heard of third class vapors (or second class vapors for that matter), but I suspected that Eric had something to do with the strange greasy stains on the wall, and wasn't prepared to admit it. With further questioning we got to the bottom of things and my suspicions proved correct. Even four-year olds are fast to blame others for their own actions. No wonder we have problems trying to reclaim our economy, our schools, and our environment. The problem is most of us are unprepared or reluctant to assume responsibility for our actions.

I think it was Thomas Jefferson who said that a democracy was impossible without educated citizens. More recently it was the leader who turned around S.A.S. Airlines, Jan Carlzon who observed that without information employees cannot take responsibility, and with it they can do nothing *but* take responsibility. Responsibility comes from having information. It's hard to have one without the other.

Few want to assume responsibility. If Richard Nixon had just admitted it was his fault (leadership), or if the president of Exxon had admitted that it was his fault (lack of enforced standards), we would have viewed both differently. But when we can see and smell the smoking pistol and encounter denial, we are especially unforgiving!

Many of the burdens we place on our enormous government bureaucracy are the result of citizens unwilling to take responsibility. Since I don't expect to see a dime of the money I'm submitting for social security, I am forced to assume responsibility for my own financial security upon retirement. Countless laws are passed and require enforcement because we are unwilling to assume responsibility for our actions. Everything from littering, bankruptcy, child support, and the mandated use of seat belts to the types of containers we can store gasoline for our lawn mowers are described by some law.

Do these laws assure that we'll buckle up for that short drive to the grocery store and avoid unsafe gasoline containers? Probably not. You can't seem to legislate common sense and personal responsibility. Oh, we can punish those we catch, but repeat offenders, from drunken driving to rape, have become something of a cliché. Even extreme forms of punishment seem ineffective in imparting a sense of responsibility.

When Magic Johnson announced his HIV infection and assumed responsibility for his actions, his respect and impact soared. When football player Lyle Alzado assumed responsibility for his actions and admitted his brain cancer was the likely result of his use of illegal steroids, we admired his courage, even though the consequences were tragic. It's easy to accept responsibility for our successes, but it is more difficult to accept responsibility for our failures or shortcomings.

One of the great challenges you have working with patients, is helping them assume responsibility for their conditions and mentoring them to make informed health care decisions in the future. The most successful at this are doctors who have high patient visit averages (PVA). This statistic, also known as "retention", is derived by taking the total number of monthly visits divided by the number of new patients that month. This approximation, while not perfectly accurate,is much more practical than going through all the patient files and counting the number of visits since they began care. Because it has the result of an averaging effect, months in which there is a significant influx of new patients send the figure downward. Likewise, when the number of new patients is down, the figure advances upward. Each monthly PVA should be averaged with the preceding eleven months to give you a more accurate idea of whether you're moving up or down.

Offices that have high PVA share several things in common:

1. Excellent communication skills: Patient education is a cornerstone of these types of offices. Appropriate patient education gives patients a complete understanding of the full nature and severity of their conditions. Without this appreciation, patients do not return to the office after their symptoms disappear. Patient education is critical.

2. Outgoing personalities: Everyone with patient contact in these offices is outgoing and clearly excited about chiropractic. Their passion is contagious and it makes them attractive for patients to be around. These doctors quickly build rapport and avoid scolding patients when they miss appointments or admit they're not doing their exercises. Patients find their enthusiasm and openness compelling.

3. Fast and effective adjusting procedures: Because these offices are even more responsible than their patients, they respect the patients' time. Patients are taught they are buying the doctor's talent, not the doctor's time. Patients meet a doctor who is ready to listen, but focused and relatively uninterested in Aunt Martha's car troubles or last night's televised awards program.

4. A team mentality: What's really remarkable in offices with high retention figures is the way they treat their staff. Ask staff members what they do and invariably they say they work "with" doctor SoAndSo, not "for" doctor SoAndSo. Big difference! This also translates into lower turnover, higher job satisfaction, and a career orientation. How can you expect patients to stay, if you can't even *pay* your staff to hang around?

5. High levels of self-esteem: Self-esteem is the undercurrent of all successful marriages, successful families, and successful offices. With adequate amounts of self-esteem these doctors are quick to regularly question the status quo, implement change, and look for better ways of doing things. When they make a mistake they willingly admit it (take responsibility) and blame themselves when the stats turn downward— not the staff, the weather, the insurance companies, or other outside influences.

6. Ability to run a business: Regardless of how good an adjuster you are, if you can't run a business, your ability to share your valuable skills and make an impact in your community is severely reduced. These doctors create systems and document them clearly in procedure manuals, so everyone's attention can be on the more important aspects of patient care, patient communications, and patient motivation instead of handling exceptions and dealing with the latest emergency.

7. Long term view of the future: All of these offices plan to be in business for many years. None are looking for a quick financial killing, early retirement, or career change. With this long-range outlook they are less bothered by patients who refuse to take responsibility and drop out of care prematurely. They congratulate the patient for considering chiropractic and make sure the patient knows they are always welcome back should their condition return (which is highly likely). Many offices report that it may take some patients as many as three or four times of beginning and then discontinuing care before they finally understand chiropractic well enough to assume the responsibility necessary for a chiropractic lifestyle. What's the hurry?

You can only assume responsibility when you are willing to search for and acknowledge cause instead of being distracted by symptom. The number of new patients you get is a symptom. How long they stay with you is a symptom. High turnover at the front desk is a symptom. Patients not "getting it" is a symptom. When patients don't refer others it's a symptom. When you're having fun in the service of others—that's a symptom too. Until you and your patients trust each other enough to recognize the cause, you are destined to repeat the frustrations of the past. Getting to the cause not only encourages responsibility, it makes each of us more responsive. ■

THE MAGIC PILL

Well, they finally developed what every chiropractor has wanted. Due to popular demand and the constant badgering of researchers, a new practice management tool has been developed that every doctor will want. Fortunately it is modestly priced and well within the financial means of virtually every chiropractic doctor. Even recent graduates can afford to buy and use this powerful practice enhancer.

Just look at what this new device can do. When used as instructed, it results in 100% patient compliance. Imagine, being able to look a patient in the eye and proposing a complete relief, rehabilitative, and wellness care treatment package and getting instant acceptance, approval, and perfect follow through! Not only do patients comply, but they are on time for their appointments and never object to rush hour waiting. When this practice enhancer is used, asking patients to bring in their spouses and children results in total participation. Referrals? Ask and you receive. Finally the practice of your dreams.

Upon further reflection I think you wouldn't wish this scenario upon your worst enemy! Remember King Midas?

Let's say you're a tennis player. Several times a week you find a court and play as many games as you can. In fact, it's the cornerstone of your exercise program. As you watch your game improve and become an increasingly better player, winning the game is not as important as a challenging volley. You're working on your form, refining your backhand, and handling the net better. Your sense of personal progress is important and you seek out players of equal skill level to keep you challenged.

Then something happens. Close matches aren't as much fun. You've reached a plateau. It's difficult to find anyone challenging enough. After reaching a certain skill level, winning becomes more important. Almost a preoccupation. It seems a constant battle to find players to challenge you. The games you lose become burned in your mind. "I should've..." "I could've..." Instead of enjoying the game, winning becomes the goal. In fact, many of your friends observe how you've changed and they're not as interested in playing with you as they were before.

Over drinks at the juice bar at the club where you frequently play, a friend asks you if you've heard about the latest surefire winning strategy. You perk up. "It guarantees that you win every time," your friend explains.

"What is it?" you ask. "How much does it cost?" "Does it work?"

"Oh sure," your friend reassures. "When you use this simple technique you win every time. You become a winning machine."

"How do I get one," you ask, as your pulse quickens and you try to hide your enthusiasm.

"Well, it's really quite simple," your friend smiles, "you just play seven year-olds. You win every time!"

The point? Personal satisfaction and fulfillment come from something other than reaching a statistic or the achievement of some arbitrary goal you've set. Too many doctors think practice is a destination instead of a process. "I'll be happy when..." "I'll be successful when..." "If I could just..." Those that are having the most fun in chiropractic recognize practice is a process, not a destination. You never "get there." The objective is to keep the game going. When you win, you actually lose. You lose your excitement. You lose your vision. You lose the fun that practice should be. One hundred percent compliance would be boring and you would quickly lose interest in chiropractic.

Doctors who wisely acknowledge this reality are unfazed by changes in the worker's compensation or personal injury laws in their state. They are in touch with reality and recognize fewer patients have insurance and they develop strategies to deal with it. Do they fight for equality and

104

support their state association's legislative action committee? Of course. The key point is that they admit times are changing and will continue to change. The joy is in the process, not in finally getting somewhere and reaching a certain practice volume. Because there will always be someone faster, bigger, or better than you.

This is not a dress rehearsal. If you're not having fun or you're not enjoying the process of educating and caring for patients and stimulating them to bring in others, you have several choices:

Change careers: Does the grass look greener somewhere else? If your heart isn't in chiropractic and you think you can serve others in a different capacity, go for it. I know several doctors in various stages of transition now. Do their practices suffer? Sure. Make sure your profession serves you to the same degree it allows you to serve others. If you feel obligated only because of your education or out of duty to your mortgage payments, stop killing yourself! Unless of course your idea of a great tombstone is, "He never missed a payment."

Start over: This is a common approach, particularly among the more entrepreneurial chiropractors. Sell the practice and move somewhere else and start over. For those who enjoy the adrenalin-pumping days of start up and dislike the maintenance of a "business," this may be a viable solution. Do remember though, you'll take the problem patients, the problem procedures, and the problem business skills with you wherever you go. That's fine, just remember to enjoy the process. You'll never have the perfect practice.

Sabotage the practice: This is a favorite among those who find selling the practice and starting over too risky. Instead, they test the practice. To use the earlier tennis metaphor, they become the Bobby Riggs of chiropractic. They try to practice with the equivalent of one hand tied behind their backs. They try it without patient education. They try it without any staff. They try it by practicing only two days a week. They try it while trying to build a building. Or they try it while dividing their interest between their political role in the state association and some pyramid marketing scheme.

Change your attitude: This may be the healthiest, yet the most difficult to achieve. Someone once said that the reasonable man tries to change himself, whereas the unreasonable man tries to change the world.

When you enjoy the process of practicing chiropractic and of changing one patient at a time, you're changing the world. It may not be dramatic or instantly obvious to the rest of the world, but your community is not the same.

When you are no longer focused by a purpose larger than yourself, burnout and self doubt can take hold. In a recent interview comedian Chevy Chase observed his lost passion for civil rights, the Vietnam war, women's rights and other issues. "Those were great days. It saddens me to think that there's something I'm missing, something that I've lost, and I wonder what I traded it for. I miss the passion."

Since the beginning, chiropractic has been a profession of Lone Rangers, individualists who embraced a healing art they were told didn't work and no one wanted. If chiropractic becomes too easy and too accepted and the battle seems too predictable, then chiropractic might surely be in trouble! Are you ready to go to jail for chiropractic like generations of chiropractors before you? Are you willing to publicly take a stand for chiropractic? Are you walking the talk?

Our bodies are continuums that grow and age and die. One's understanding of chiropractic is a continuum that goes from unawareness to unconscious competence. And certainly practice is a continuum from start up to retirement. What's the hurry? Enjoy the journey. ■

ON BECOMING
A COACH

I bet this isn't an exciting time for practice management firms. The good old days of plentiful insurance money has been replaced by an increasingly competitive environment in which fewer and fewer patients have insurance and those that do, have sky high deductibles. What chiropractors have discovered is that the A.M.A. wasn't the enemy, it was the "sickness care" orientation of the insurance industry! The world has changed, and few practice management firms have kept up.

Sadly, most practice management firms are still beating the dead horse of insurance. Supplying "super-duper-can't-fail" narratives and complicated insurance procedures to increase the likelihood of getting paid is simply rearranging the deck chairs on the Titanic.

Since hope springs eternal, some are placing their future in the hands of legislators who will lead us into some type of nationalized/socialized health care (actually sickness care) system for all citizens. "Like they have in Canada," they proclaim. Have you talked to any Canadian chiropractors? In Ontario it's called 22 visit-itis. In British Columbia it's 12 visits, without reimbursement for X-rays. Even in light of the Wilk case, the RAND Corporation study, and the *20/20* story, chiropractic care is likely to be capped, severely limited, or shortchanged in some way. Even in the best case scenario, income from third-party payers will never be like it was in the early 1980s. Let's do what we can with the legislatures and national lobbying, but the wishful thinking of most practitioners is not likely to materialize.

Practice management firms have played a valuable role in the profession by helping countless doctors recognize that they are at the helm of a small business, and not merely drug-free healers. Recent advancements and sophistication in the chiropractic profession are partly due to the efforts of a handful of reputable management specialists. Yet the tactics they've taught during the last 10 to 12 years are less effective today. The notion that you can control patients into compliance or manage them into doing the right thing is a thing of the past. The generation showing up in chiropractic offices these days has changed all that.

Teaching doctors and their staff to be confrontive and authoritarian in their patient management is no longer effective. This authoritarian, "do as I say" approach may work during the early stages of care when patients are experiencing painful symptoms, but its effect is counter-productive later as they feel better. The compliance in the beginning is accompanied by the same resentment we feel about government red tape, the mind-numbing experience at the Department of Motor Vehicles, or the long, unexplained delays on the runway before take off. Patients resent being "talked down to" and ordered around as if they can't think for themselves. Baby boomers, like their four-year old children have a propensity to want to know "why." Unless you anticipate this "tell-me-why" mindset you are prone to poor compliance, poor word-of-mouth advertising, and less than optimal patient rapport.

Why do I need X-rays? Why can't you do something to help me on my first visit? Why do I have to "sign in"? Why do I have to see a video? Why to I have to take my clothes off? Why do I feel worse than when I came here? Why does a four-minute adjustment cost so much? Why won't my insurance company pay for this? Why can't you prescribe drugs? Why don't you work more closely with the medical profession? Why do you treat children? Why do I need to keep coming back? Why?

This unspoken predisposition to want to know why is hard for some doctors to accept because many patients are not verbal or self-confident enough to even confront a doctor with these questions. They are relieved when the information is volunteered without asking for it, or they'll ask your staff instead. Don't be fooled into thinking that just because they don't ask some of these questions that they are mindless robots, ready to obey every instruction!

No, the old dictatorial, authoritarian bedside manner of the past no longer works with the today's new patients. More appropriate is the doctor as a health care "mentor" or "coach." Coaching is an entirely different orientation. In some ways it is easier than being the all-knowing-omniscient doctor of the past. And in other ways it is much more challenging. Rarely do coaches get the instant gratification that dictators enjoy. Plus, it can be especially frustrating for doctors with years of clinical experience to see patients squander their health potential by ignoring suggested lifestyle modifications or visit frequency recommendations.

Besides taking a burden off your shoulders (that to a patient you didn't ever really have), being a coach requires a new way of thinking. If you want to be a better coach to your patients, here are some ideas to consider:

Sense of team: Being a coach automatically connotes a sense of teamwork. For a team to be effective there must be leadership from the coach and mutual respect for the "players." It also suggests that each individual has a certain set of responsibilities. Make sure your patients know what you and your staff are willing to do, as you help them recover their health, and what you expect of them. Chiropractic has always been a partnership approach to health. It shouldn't be something that "just happens" *to* a patient. It happens *with* a patient.

Teach the fundamentals: This is where patient education comes in. Not only does a coach explain the rules of the game, players depend upon the coach to teach the basics—everything from how to grip the bat, kick the ball, or throw a pass. In the health care arena this means explaining the function of the nervous system, how the body heals, and acquainting patients with the basics of physiology. Most patients are merely guests in their own bodies and have no idea how it functions. Always go back to the basics—it's what makes chiropractic make so much sense!

Have a game plan: Every player needs to know your strategy. What's the line up? What can we expect? What are some areas of concern? If you want patients to abandon their limited notions of health, you must share your vision so they can understand and respond appropriately. Strategies change throughout the season and throughout each individual game (visit). Keep patients in the dark and they become powerless to contribute. Share your plan and watch compliance improve.

Set an example: How's your own health these days? What's your physical fitness plan? What are you doing besides getting regular chiropractic care to maintain good health? Rarely do you find patients who are healthier than their doctor. When patients reach your level of health, or that of your staff, they are prompted to drop out. Coaches lead by example. Don't confuse this with the "healthier-than-thou" attitude some doctors project! Leading by example is quiet and non-judgmental. When the coach has high standards it's more likely players will set high standards, too.

Praise: This is one of the more difficult mindsets to overcome. There was a time when you could order patients to comply or scare patients into submission. That's unsportsman-like conduct. Coaches must continually encourage their players to set ever higher goals and levels of achievement. And while every coach's style is different, find a behavior you want repeated and praise it! Want patients to do their exercises at home? Lavish praise in celebration of their discipline. Praise patients for keeping their appointments, showing up on time, bringing their spouses to reports, referring others, and other conduct you want to encourage. What gets rewarded, gets done.

Heads up: This is one of the other important roles of a coach: watching for shifts in the wind or changes on the playing field that might necessitate a change in strategy. Coaches need to be sensitive to backsliding, or off-handed remarks that may reveal internal struggle or doubts that may sabotage performance. Similarly, coaches look for opportunities to ask questions, talking about the health of other family members, and other occasions that reveal clues about issues that may influence compliance or referrals.

Celebrate: The best coaches make the game fun to play. Yet, if the coach isn't having fun, the players probably aren't either. If financial pressures, staff management problems, or a lack of energy or purpose are hobbling the coach, the players are affected. Your game plan should identify certain goals or milestones on a patient's road to recovery. Celebrate when they are reached! Compliment the patient in front of others. Send an encouraging letter or card. Take his or her picture. Let the rest of your "team" see your Most Valuable Player.

Those who have ever coached a little league team know that coaching is an entirely different way of thinking than that of a dictator. For those who were "ordered around" as children or are accustomed to being spoon fed by others, becoming a coach can be an exciting growth opportunity. Doctors who have created a successful practice using the old methods of the past are likely to find coaching difficult and uncomfortable. It's hard to argue with years of experience and cabinets bulging with patient files from the past. But that was a different time. Welcome to the future!

It's unlikely that chiropractors will fully assume the role of being coaches until the examples set by management firms reflect this new attitude. In the same way doctors can't "manage" patients, management firms can't "manage" doctors. The awareness of this fundamental shift can encourage responsibility and increase a doctor's self-esteem sufficiently to propel chiropractic into its second hundred years. ■

THE CHIROPRACTIC
PERFORMANCE

One of the most compelling reasons for efficient management skills and the implementation of a business "system" in your office is, it allows for a better chiropractic performance for your patients. Many chiropractic doctors fail to realize that the performance; the set up, delivery, and bedside manner, is equally, or more important than the adjustment itself. Proper office management allows more attention and focus on the performance of chiropractic.

Unfortunately, some doctors approach the adjusting table with the same amount of thought as the zealous cook, who discovers half way through mixing a cake that a key ingredient is missing. Not only does this sabotage a new patient's perception of chiropractic, it can devalue an established patient's care. In fact, I'd venture to guess that a less-than-optimal spinal manipulation, if rendered as a magnificent performance, can be perceived by the patient as better than a more specific chiropractic adjustment delivered by a doctor who seems detached, distant, or preoccupied. The performance is an often overlooked part of the psychological component of the healing process.

The impact of this shortcoming is especially apparent in the offices of doctors who are not particularly expressive or outgoing. These are often analytical types who have invested heavily in technique seminars, are voracious readers, and have overlooked the "art" of chiropractic and focused instead on the "science" of chiropractic. These doctors are often so focused on their adjusting technique, that the sometimes more important psychological needs of the patient are neglected. The result is a perfectly rendered adjustment on a patient who perceives the doctor as uninterested and uncommunicative. With a lack of communication from the doctor the patient fills in the blanks, interpreting the event in their own terms. They may incorrectly think their case is difficult, that they are not responding as expected, or worse, that the doctor is unsure. This "poor performance" (as perceived by the patient) sabotages an optimum doctor/patient relationship.

The performance here is more than just impeccable bedside (table-side) manners. It has many component parts. An entire book could be written about each part. Until then, here are some ideas you might want to consider as you evaluate your chiropractic performance and look for possible ways of improving it:

Personality: If you know you're not a great communicator, start working on it! It is the single most important aspect of your performance. Doctors who regularly do lectures or welcome public speaking opportunities almost always have better practices. In fact, the common denominator of every successful practice, regardless of how you define success, is a doctor who is a good communicator. You may have to leave your comfort zone. You cannot remain a spectator. Get in the game and test your beliefs, test your values, and share your vision. Confront your greatest fear. Make some mistakes. Grow!

Preparation: What is your plan to fully utilize the opportunity presented by having patients in your office—an environment you control? What impression or outcome do you want today's patients to leave with? What is your purpose for being in practice? What specific action steps will you need to take to better assure the fulfillment of your purpose?

Preparation means you'll need a plan (and a back up) to accomplish your purpose. Magnificent performances don't just happen, they are well thought out. When a musician or gourmet chef gives a concert or makes an exotic dessert preparation look easy, it's because they were totally prepared. They visualized the exact outcome or effect they wanted (not what they didn't want) and their performance was conducted on a more powerful unconscious level.

If you are already practicing on an unconscious level, the challenge is what you do to prevent your synergistic flow of total focus from becoming a boring routine. Yet, this is when you can truly give more attention to your verbal and non-verbal communication in the adjusting room. Set up a video camera to record what happens tableside. Compare the energy and focus at 10:30 A.M. with 5:30 P.M.

First impression: If you've heard the classic line that "your appearance is speaking so loudly I can't hear what you're saying," you know the importance of a first impression. This happens all the time in chiropractic offices. The first impression starts with the quality of any outside marketing efforts (yellow pages) and the location of your office (is the neighborhood on the way up or the way down?) to opening the door to your reception room. Walk in the front door of your office. What's the first thing your eye goes to?

Apprehensive patients size up your office very critically because they figure you had a hand in creating its tone. It serves as a metaphor of the quality of care they think will be rendered in the back room.

Patients gauge the staff and doctor in the same way. This isn't an excuse to be extravagant (unless maybe you practice in Beverly Hills), however invest in quality office furnishings and clothing. Don't expect to see white collar "influencers" of your community consulting your office if you're still wearing polyester! Dress just one notch above your average patient or the type of patient you want. Your appearance, office resources, and increased capacity come first, then the patients come. You cannot perform at your best with an adjusting table you don't like or X-ray equipment the produces unpredictable results.

Audience: The audience is an important component of any performance. The key to any extraordinary doctor/patient interaction is a thorough understanding of the audience. I remember having a seminar audience turn on me in Mt. Horeb, Wisconsin. I was invited to speak on the subject of patient education to alumni and students practicing the Gonstead adjusting technique. Since most new patients could care less which adjusting technique the doctor uses, I didn't give any thought to the anterior adjustments shown in a patient education video tape I was demonstrating at the time!

Knowing your audience goes beyond acknowledging the patient's symptomatic complaint and assuring them you think you can help. On a more powerful level it means to anticipate their concerns. How are they going to be feeling and what are they going to be thinking when they are completing your admitting forms? What's going through their minds as they hear the drop piece on your adjusting table? How much is this going to cost? How long is this going to take? Will it hurt? Will I have to keep coming back for the rest of my life? The internal dialogue goes on and on. Doctors who recognize this voice and volunteer answers (without the patient having to ask!) build strong bridges of rapport that later translate into trust and better compliance.

Timing: Ask any comedian what is most important part of their performance is and they'll tell you, timing. What else can explain the difference between an "I died out there" performance and an "I killed them" performance using the same material?

How many times have you rushed your report, knowing the reception room was filling up? How many times have you dismissed a patient's intimate revelations? How many times have you cut off a staff member's meandering explanation of a problem to "cut to the chase"? Timing is everything. The key is to have the rapport necessary to match the patient's pacing.

Delivery: Patients look to the doctor for cues as to the proper patient "etiquette" during the actual adjustment. Should I close my eyes? Do I talk during the adjustment? If you're going to tango make sure you lead and you tell your partner (patient) what kind of dance you'll be dancing.

Patients look to the doctor for cues as to how to judge the importance of an adjustment. If you believe it is paramount, and you want patients to believe similarly, talking about the Lakers game while delivering a cervical rotation is probably inappropriate. So is gum chewing, humming along with piped-in Karen Carpenter singing "We've Only Just Begun", and other behavior that would indicate a lack of present time consciousness.

The punch line: If after every adjustment your brain produces the sound of thunderous applause, let your patients in on the performance. Praise patients, "You did great!" Educate patients, "Now you have better range of motion!" Motivate patients, "That ought to shave a few more strokes off your game!" Future pace your patients, "Now you'll be able to lift those grandchildren of yours!" It's not so much what you say, it's how you say it. Patients want to sense passion, excitement, and a sense of culmination.

Feedback loops: Part of the performance must include some type of monitoring so the doctor can keep tabs on the relationship. "How are we doing?" Every adjustment with every patient may be your very last. You can't be sure that any patient will ever return again. Part of the performance must include simple questions that can help serve to reveal their commitment and satisfaction. "How was that adjustment compared to the approach I used on Monday?" "Are afternoons still the best time for your appointments?" These and other questions can be asked without assuming a defensive posture or seeming insecure. They are casual, off-handed remarks that project self-confidence and an almost, "I-already-know-the-answer" attitude. Yet, questions like these can create an opportunity for patients to voice a concern or express a frustration that can be remedied before it's too late.

In medicine, a placebo can be part of a performance. Its use acknowledges the important role the brain plays in the healing process. Same with chiropractic. An engaging tableside manner projects confidence and honors the patient's psychological needs. And while chiropractic is so powerful that even the crudest forms of manipulation can offer pain relief, it is the artist who multiplies the effect by his or her performance that takes patients to a higher plane of wellness. That's what patients really want: more goose bumps. The same kind they get when hearing Mariah Carey hit a high note or watching Michael Jordan fly! ■

BEDSIDE
MANNERS

It is unlikely that Doctors of Chiropractic will ever be replaced by computers or some high-tech, pneumatic-driven, robotic manipulation machine. The delivery of quality chiropractic care will almost always require the training, intuition, and creativity that only the complex human mind is capable of providing. While a certain level of job security is afforded in this observation, this security can easily be sabotaged by a doctor's lack of social skills, poor rapport-building techniques, flawed communications, or unattractive personality. These non-clinical aspects of providing patient care create one's "bedside manner." In chiropractic we might call it one's "tableside manner." This is the personality purposely projected to, or inadvertently perceived by, patients during the consultation, examination, and day-to-day adjusting procedures in your office. It holds back a great many otherwise excellent chiropractic clinicians.

Certainly personality is an important aspect of building a successful practice. Ask any doctor who has attempted to duplicate the results taught by many practice management specialists who were themselves dynamic practitioners. Many of these procedures make sense only when they are combined with the originating personality. Without it, the procedure or communication model becomes an empty shell and takes on the appearance of a gimmick or an insincere form of patient manipulation. Chiropractic delivered without a personality is like watching television without the sound. It lacks depth and character.

It's unlikely personality transplants will ever be perfected.

Some claim that fundamental personality development occurs by age six or seven. Isn't it the Jesuits who say, "Give me a child for his first six years and I'll own him for the rest of his life"? Does that mean you're hopelessly stuck with your current personality forever? I don't think so. People can change. I've seen it happen.

In the years I've done seminars and conducted in-office consultations, I've met countless doctors with attractive bedside manners. Here are some common denominators which describe these most successful doctors.

Energy: Doctors with effective bedside manners have a high level of two different types of energy. Their psychological energy translates into passion for what they do. They communicate their high level of commitment by this enthusiasm. The other type of energy is physical energy. They have endurance and stamina so they don't tire easily. They are doers. They're still going strong at the end of the day and have the capacity to devote still more energy to their family. They are at their proper weight and, simply put, are quite healthy themselves.

Action step: Become passionate about your work. Find others who are passionate and discover what "revs" them up. Confront your greatest fear about your technique. Take a few post X-rays to confirm that the application of your technique is making structural changes. Start a work out program. Get fit. You must become healthier than your average patient!

Rapport: Doctors with responsive patients who refer others are skillful in establishing rapport with patients. These doctors get along equally well with time-conscious Type A personalities, skeptics, grandmothers, and uncooperative children. Their versatility projects a nonjudgmental atmosphere in which all types of patients feel comfortable and welcome.

Action step: Come closer to matching the pace set by your patients. If they speak quickly, you speak quickly. Match their use of language by listening carefully to their cues. Do they make decisions based on facts or feelings? Make sure you speak their decision-making language.

Accept patients for who they are. Assume the role of a coach and a mentor. Avoid the "healthier-than-thou" or "do-as-I-say" posture that is so tempting. Be thankful they have entered your sphere of influence. Celebrate their success. Congratulate and affirm their positive behavior such as keeping their appointments, doing their exercises, referring others, etc. Smile.

Time: These doctors run on time. They are keenly aware that a patient's time is valuable, too. Not only is the day well-planned and organized, the doctor is in a "real time" consciousness. He or she knows what time it is and is focused on the moment. This doesn't come off as a rushed form of preoccupation. Just the reverse. Because of good scheduling and a clear purpose, the doctor can truly "be with" the patient in mind and body. Patients sense this focused presence and it raises their self-esteem and makes them feel important.

Action step: Run on time. Don't allow walk-in patients to sabotage the relationships you have with your more considerate patients. Teach your staff proper scheduling to avoid conflicts with reports, new patients, and routine adjusting by color-coding patient's names in the appointment book. Make sure your patients know they are buying your skills, not the time they spend with you. Realize your patients have a life and that chiropractic isn't its focus!

Communication: The best practices are run by the best communicators. The more esoteric your adjusting technique, the more responsibility you assume to explain it and generally over-communicate with your patients. An organized and systematic patient education program is just the start. These doctors jump at the chance to talk about chiropractic to groups and regularly conduct lay lectures and orientation sessions for their new patients. Patients know where their doctor stands on a variety of health issues and they find his or her knowledge and openness to be quite appealing.

Action steps: If you do leg length checks tell the patient which leg is longer or shorter. On every visit! Volunteer information in advance. Use language the patient can understand. Don't wait for the patient to ask. Assume every patient wants to know what you're thinking today. Because they do. Keep a running database of what patients tell you on their travel card or SOAP notes so you can refer to these topics on subsequent visits.

Appearance: It may not be fair, but our first and most lasting impression of someone is formed in the first three to five seconds. Successful doctors are sensitive to this fact and are extremely aware of their personal appearance. Their clothing is fashionably current without being faddish. They project an optimistic, upbeat outlook with a polished, button-down attention to detail. They wear natural fabrics, avoid polyester, and have their 100% cotton shirts and blouses professionally laundered.

Action steps: Plan to consistently look a notch better than your typical patient. Men should consider the cost of earrings, a Mr. T. neck chain starter kit, and trendy accessories on the image they project. Make sure your breath always passes muster. Have regular manicures—your hands are your scalpel. Pay extra for good looking comfortable shoes and make sure they're polished. Wash your hands frequently throughout the day so you don't inadvertently transfer a patient's perfume or cologne to someone else, communicating a lack of cleanliness. If you're still smoking, stop. Breath mints don't cover up the odor.

Purpose: This is the most important. Having a clear understanding of one's purpose can compensate for many other shortcomings in one's bedside manner. Doctors who lack the charm and communication skills of an outgoing personality, yet have tapped into the universal power of recognizing their purpose, have a distinct edge. What is your purpose for being in chiropractic? What would you do if money were no object and you were certain to succeed? What would you do if they outlawed chiropractic?

Action steps: Get in touch with your fundamental purpose for being in chiropractic. Take a stand. Make a list of the reasons why you decided to get into chiropractic in the first place. Recall the idealism and optimism you had in chiropractic college. What would it take to rekindle it? Find a mentor who's doing what you'd like to be doing or has a practice like you'd like to have. Pick his or her brain.

You are an extremely attractive and interesting person. You must be, if you were called to chiropractic! Only extraordinary people get involved in a profession they were told no one wants. It is only the rare, discerning individual who constantly seeks the truth and is comfortable with it. Your mission is to take the risk necessary to discover who you really are and make sure it is communicated to your patients. You must be a living testimonial to the value and quality of a chiropractic lifestyle. Are you hiding your lamp under a bowl? ■

ESCAPING
THE COCOON

From the personality tests I've taken I know that I occupy the quadrant commonly called the "Analytical" or the "Thinker." I've been branded as an individual that tends to weigh the facts when making decisions and is less "emotive" than others. Somehow I became a person that attempts to gather all the facts before going forward. How I became this person or adopted this approach to life, I am not yet certain. And while those who make poor impulse decisions may value the methodical, thought-provoking way I make decisions, it wasn't until recently that I discovered the myopia that my orientation lends to my world view.

Merrill and Reid, the authors of *Personal Styles and Effective Performance* outline four personality quadrants, Analytical (thinking), Amiable (relationship), Driver (action), and Expressive (intuition). Most of us find ourselves using one of these four styles more than the others in the process of living of our lives. Some of us put a lot of value on how we feel (Expressive) about a particular topic when making decisions. Others make decisions and then later count the costs (Driver). Still others look to the relationships (Amiable) involved when making decisions. And then there are those of us who weigh the facts (Analytical). This orientation significantly shapes our world view, our habits, and our ability to communicate effectively with others.

In the chiropractic profession, the most successful doctors seem to fall into the Expressive quadrant. Their outgoing styles and sensitivity equip them to better communicate their clinical goals and objectives to patients. Patients are extremely responsive to this open conduit. They feel at ease and are more likely to trust someone who is perceived as open, available, and obviously committed to their chiropractic decision.

Doctors who seem to have the most difficulty are those in the Analytical quadrant. Because of the way they value facts and are relentless seekers of the truth, they attend countless technique seminars and are always looking for the best ways to care for their patients. On the corner of their desks can be found countless clinical journals and publications littered with the latest reports and blind studies of this or that. Analyticals commit inordinate amounts of time in a constant search for objectivity and accountability. Their clinical excellence is legendary. Since they are constantly searching for the truth, they often inadvertently tune out the patient. Combined with their lack of obvious emotion, many patients see them as insensitive, distant, or consumed with other matters.

Their reserved show of emotion or constant "internal dialogue" can appear as a sense of tentativeness or cautiousness that raises concerns, even doubts, in the minds of sensitive patients. Because patients often interpret a lack of outward enthusiasm and confidence as disinterest, a doctor's analytical personality style can interfere with a patients' need for reassurance and confidence.

Are doctors of a certain personality profile likely to be more successful? Probably. In the same way Amiables seem to make great caregivers and take charge Drivers seem to make better leaders. Our personalities can give us a head start toward success in our chosen field. Can people change? Sure. Yet in stress or a time of crisis, we often resort to our fundamental and predisposed personalities.

When audiences attend a seminar, witness a speech, or attend one of my presentations, they are often surprised to learn that I was the Analytical high school "wallflower." Certainly I am living proof that people can change!

I pride myself in being open and confident enough to actively solicit questions during my presentations. I prefer the interruption because a question from the audience (patients) is a valuable form of feedback. When an audience takes on the inanimate features of Mount Rushmore, I get concerned!

Fortunately, the most disarming, caught-me-off-balance question I ever received wasn't during, but after a seminar in Ohio, from a doctor who, I had noticed, was lingering towards the back of the room. As I was arranging my notes and preparing to leave the room, he came forward. He had this introspective look on his face and his silence and flat emotional response (Analytical) during the day-long session, would normally have led me to believe that he was not enjoying the seminar.

"You mentioned today that the best offices were run by the best communicators," he ventured tentatively, capsulizing the essence of a full three hour presentation. "How does one become a good communicator like you?"

For the first time in a long time I was caught off guard. He had asked a question that was in some ways more pertinent than much of the material I had covered all day. And while I was caught off guard then, here are some ideas I wish I had shared at the time:

1. Know your purpose. Until you know why you've been put on this earth and get alignment with a vision larger than yourself, you will remain in your protective cocoon. The truly happy people I've met are bothered about something and they are often preoccupied with a cause. There are many tools and resources that can help you in the self discovery of your purpose. To be an effective communicator you must have a purpose.

2. Recognize the value of performance. Patients and seminar attendees want to see a doctor and speaker charged up and passionate. Sure, patients want assistance with the healing process and seminar goers have paid for quality information. These expectations are usually fulfilled quickly. The rapport and trust needed for long term relationships must come from obviously communicated confidence and excitement. Once you acknowledge that chiropractic is a performance, you'll discover a new and fulfilling level of therapeutics that transcends the introduction of appropriate thrust along fixated joint planes!

3. Get strength from criticism. The best communicators recognize the importance of feedback loops for confirming that their message is being received and decoded properly. By acquiring the necessary clinical expertise, it is easy to take a non-defensive position when the inevitable criticism arises. There's no need to be "right" all the time. Anyway, it's just somebody's opinion!

4. Know your stuff. It goes without saying that the best in every field have their information down cold. Confidence comes from routinely taking post X-rays. Call the patient after the first adjustment. Confront your most terrifying clinical fears. If you want the confidence to go boldly, know your "stuff." Know your limits too! Know when to refer out.

5. Face your greatest fear. Are you one of those who thinks there is such a thing as "security"? Are you afraid what the other doctors in your town will think? Who are you trying to impress? What would you do if they came and took away all your toys? Would your family still love you? Are you postponing the inevitable? Clean up your relationships. Clean out your closets. Be at ease with the world you've created.

6. Get out of your cocoon. Somewhere inside you might be a hurting little boy or girl. Someone who could be happily occupied for hours in the woods, by a creek, or in the backyard sandbox. Was this beautiful child hurt by a smothering mother or an emotionally distant father? Come out of your cocoon. This is your life. Take a deep breath. Soar like a butterfly. Set yourself free! Become!

So while I've learned to be more emotive, I still do it in a somewhat analytical fashion. Sometimes I have to pretend I'm excited about my work. When I have to pretend, I know I've lost sight of the big picture. And then the passion and commitment all come back.

You can change . . . if you want to. ■

DISCIPLINING
THE DOCTOR

"Spare the rod, spoil the child," goes the old adage. Disciplining a child is considered one of the highest forms of love by the writers of *Proverbs*. But the discipline missing in chiropractic isn't the punishment given patients for their poor spinal hygiene or missed appointments. It's the doctor's discipline in setting a good example and being an excellent specimen of good health. I can hear it on the telephone when doctors call and I can see it on doctors at seminars. And patients see it too. You're out of shape!

Forget about elaborate new patient procedures. Ignore a new incentive plan for your staff. Abandon your new affordable fees. And you might as well give up your plans for a family practice of well patients. Because if you're out of shape physically or mentally, besides setting a poor example, you don't have the energy necessary to inspire patients or your staff. In the same way you've become lethargic, so has your practice. For many doctors the stats have to take a nose dive or the staff has to mutiny before corrective action is taken. It's just like your patients. They wait until they are desperate before dialing the seven digits of your phone number. The phone numbers doctors call are more likely to be of a practice "management" company, a new seminar, or the local purveyor of airplane lessons. While these diversions may be satisfying momentarily, they treat the symptoms instead of the cause.

The cause is rarely procedural. It is almost always the doctor's mental and physical condition. It is the underlying cause of many practice-related challenges.

Mental Conditioning

When it comes to the chicken or the egg, this is the egg. This is where it all starts. If your brain is out of shape, every other aspect of your life and your practice is out of shape. Few would disagree. But how do you know if your brain is out of shape? Here are some neurological tests you can administer privately to find out:

1. What was the last good idea you came up with?
2. When was the last time you laughed so hard your side ached?
3. What was the last non-chiropractic book you read?
4. How many hours of television do you watch each week?
5. What was the last risk you took?
6. What was the last time you tried some new type of food?
7. When was the last celebration you had with your staff?
8. When was the last time you had goose bumps?
9. How much alcohol, chocolate, or potato chips are you eating?
10. How long are you sleeping each night?

It is said the most powerful aphrodisiac is the brain. Similarly, the most powerful practice aid is your brain. You can't get water from an empty pail. So if you want to be more creative, more alive, and have more fun, you've got to put new ideas in your brain. Something difficult to do pounding on backs all day, isolated in your office!

"Feed your head," warbled Grace Slick of Jefferson Airplane. But a drug-induced high isn't what's needed here! Doctors in the throes of burn out are already high on television, M & Ms, or self-pity. Caregivers such as doctors and chiropractic assistants find reclaiming their lives difficult because they are often reluctant to invest in themselves, either out of guilt or wanting to avoid a feeling of selfishness. However, without working on themselves, every other aspect of their lives and their practices remain unhealthy and out of balance. It's not a question of *whether* the investment will be made, it's simply *when*. How uncomfortable does the status quo have to get before circumstances give you the discipline necessary to heal yourself?

Here are a few ideas you might consider in the care and feeding of your brain.

Set higher standards. A common denominator among those searching for answers is they have low standards. Or worse, no standards! Set some new or higher standards for your life. How many hours of mind-numbing television will you allow yourself? How many non-chiropractic books are you going to read this month? This year? How many hours of sleep do you really need? How much family time are you reserving each day? Each week? Clean out your closets, your desk, and your life. If you have trouble being accountable to yourself, share your standards with someone who you want to "nag" you (probably not your spouse!).

Take meaningful risks. Fire walks, ropes courses, rafting trips, or bungy jumping are exotic, but the sizzle is unlikely to last but a week or two back at the office. More meaningful would be to regularly attend a local Toastmaster group. According to surveys, public speaking is considered by many to be more terrifying than death! When you confront this fear and master it, it will improve every other aspect of your practice. Guaranteed! But because you can't buy anything to show off and there aren't any high-tech buttons or gadgets involved, many instead will opt for the hypnotic seminar speakers and more visible exhibitions of risk-taking. Even if you don't want to speak to groups or do lay lectures, improved public speaking skills will skyrocket your practice.

Find a mentor. At the upper reaches of any career or accomplishment it becomes increasingly difficult for masters to find mentors. This happens to doctors, seminar speakers, and tennis pros. Someone, somewhere is always doing what you want to do faster or better. Find them. Seek them out. Ask someone to challenge you to reach higher, push harder, or help you abandon ideas and habits that no longer serve you. It's hard for your staff or your spouse to hold you accountable. Find someone who can catch you faking it or not giving 100%.

Sanction incompetence. You have stopped growing. To begin growing again you have to be willing to be "dumb again." Some chiropractors decide to launch a political career, dabble in the state association, take up hot air ballooning, start their own seminar, or open a satellite office. Yet rarely do these learning opportunities return the doctor's investment back to their patients or their practice. Instead, they distract from the focus of the practice to threaten their income or their future enough to force them to rededicate their energies. This is the Russian Roulette School of Personal Motivation.

Physical Conditioning

If your brain is healthy and you feel creative, vital, and alive, chances are your body is in good shape too. But for all too many chiropractors, the only exercise they get is walking from their parking space to the office and between three adjusting rooms. Hardly a cardiac conditioning program!

Like it or not, your physical appearance creates the first and most lasting impression of you and your practice. If you're 10 pounds on the heavy side or start wheezing after a flight of stairs, you're setting a poor example. Maybe this is why most chiropractic offices are merely pain relief centers and few patients bring in their children or remain for wellness care. A fat doctor is an incongruency that sabotages a patient's respect, compliance, and willingness to refer. It's not just unhealthy, it slows you down and reduces your capacity to serve and grow.

While the importance of being in top physical conditioning is rarely disputed, how to get the discipline necessary to make it a habit seems elusive. Because you're out of shape and don't have any energy, it makes it difficult to want to go out and work up a sweat. This conflict will not go away by postponing the start of your regular work out program or surrendering to the lack of instant gratification.

Here are some ideas you might consider implementing, that can help you and your practice by improving your physical fitness.

The buddy system. If you recognize you don't have the discipline necessary to sustain a workout program long enough for it to become a habit, enlist the motivation of some "peer pressure." Find a friend (again, probably not your spouse!) that is interested in working out and do it together. Being accountable to someone else can be helpful, especially during the early stages. Let's face it. Some days you won't want to go run around the nearby high school track. It helps to have someone else push you into doing what you know you need to do.

Buy some discipline. This is for movers and shakers who don't have the necessary discipline, don't have any friends, or can afford to hire someone to make them do the right things. Hire a coach or a personal trainer. Explain that you'll make up excuses not to work out, but that you're paying them to hold you accountable. Look in the yellow pages or ask around at a gym.

Set some goals. Virtually every new endeavor can be more successful if you have some measurable, attainable goal. Whether it's a lower resting heart rate, the ability to finish a 10K, run a marathon, or some other goal. Start small. There's no hurry. The key is to remain interested long enough until your workout is a habit and you start getting squirrelly when you miss one.

There's a myth circulating in our culture that if you work real hard long enough, you'll get to sit on the beach and enjoy exotic tropical drinks and not have to work anymore. It's just a myth. Instead, we must stop and smell the roses as we live our lives. Instead of a "serial" life like our parents who went to school, got married, worked, retired, and finally got to Hawaii, most of us are more likely to live a "cyclical" life. We are more likely to take sabbaticals, change careers, and go back to school before we ever retire. In fact, many of us will never retire. The key is balance while enjoying the process.

Remember getting your first bicycle? Once the training wheels were gone and you could ride around the neighborhood unaccompanied, your bicycle was a way to escape. With the wind whooshing past your ears and the ground blurring beneath you, you were free. You'd pump real hard to get to the top of the hill so you could coast down the other side without effort. If you're still in search of the effort-free life or the effort-free practice, remember, like your bicycle, you can only coast by going downhill! ■

CHIROPRACTIC WIMP

Maybe the Japanese were right. Americans are sloppy and lazy. When the Japanese see our union mentality, our remote garage door openers, and a large portion of our population overweight, it's easy to draw the wrong conclusions. But it does raise an interesting question, particularly in chiropractic: Can chiropractic rise above the path of least resistance? Who's doing what's right instead of what's easiest to defend? Who's making the choices that pay off in the long run in lieu of short term gain? Who's building the infrastructure needed to support continued growth, instead of what's expedient?

As I tour offices and meet more and more doctors, I've reached the conclusion that changing the direction and survivability of the profession will come from changing individual doctors. Practices are reflections of the doctor, not technique, geography, or birth order. State associations are reflections of the doctors in the state. And national organizations are reflections of the doctors in the nation. If you want to change the world, start by changing yourself.

Problem is, it's hard to change.

I'm convinced that books don't change doctors. Magazine articles don't change doctors. Seminars don't change doctors. And practice management groups don't change doctors. Oh, these resources may change one's awareness, from which personal change may blossom, but change has to come from within.

If you can't concentrate longer than 30 seconds, your practice is a cauldron of confusion and stress. If you are easily captivated by TV commercials and swayed by the latest fad, your practice lacks focus and purpose. If your brain is cluttered, so is your desk. You are your practice.

It's so convenient to blame your patients, your staff, your location, your scope of practice laws, insurance companies, or the winter storm, but the problem is really you. You probably won't hear this from the management firm that you pay thousands of dollars and who wants you to reup, but they know it's you, too.

Most of us don't change unless we have too.

How many are in unsuccessful marriages only because the status quo is less painful than the unknown of divorce? How many keep staff members who are sabotaging their practices only because finding and training someone else is too frightening or inconvenient? How many continue using the same office procedures but expect different results? Change is one of the most terrifying things any of us experience. The fact is, most of the people we surround ourselves with don't want us to change either. Most of us choose predictability over possibility. Change? Only if I have to.

Many of the things that we think and do that limit our potential are habits formed over many years. Changing these habits and making room for more resourceful activities that serve us better is difficult. Some suggest it takes as long as 40 days to form a new habit. Instead of consciously taking it upon ourselves to eliminate thoughts or replace traditions that no longer serve us, most of us wait until there's a gun to our head. We are forced to change. If you won't change on your own behalf, just wait long enough and you'll have to change to survive. Not exactly the best way to undertake a new approach!

If bottom line results are what you want, and I freely admit these words will not affect the real changes you probably want (or need), how do you change without the added pressure of changing simply to survive?

It's you. First you have to decide. Deciding to change only occurs after the awareness of the possible benefits of changing become real. Deciding to change is a quiet something that happens inside you. No one knows you've decided. You don't look different. In fact, to anyone else, you haven't changed. But once you've decided, you're more than half way there.

The next step is to take the risk and, as Nike shoe commercials suggest, "just do it." This is a big step. If "it" is something highly visible or involves others, the risk is high. What if someone sees you changing? What if you fail? What if you don't "look good?" Change may not be pretty. The self-esteem necessary to expose yourself to these possibilities is enormous. Which is one reason why most people don't change and simply allow their lives to happen to them. To change, we must first acknowledge our intrinsic worth before we recognize we are worthy of what change may bring us.

Ironically, the changes that most doctors need to make have very little to do with chiropractic. Sure, there are some simple office procedures or patient communications that can be improved, but remember the problem is the doctor. Here are some changes that you could make that might precipitate the personal breakthroughs that could result in significant changes in your practice. Some of these will sound strange, but do them and your perception will change. And change is what this is all about anyway!

1. Stop watching television. Even if all you watch is PBS with your nose cocked slightly above the horizon, abandon the "boob tube" or the "plug in drug" and find something more valuable to fill your time. You'll have to. Without putting your brain in neutral for three or four hours a day and filled with "buy-this-buy-that" commercials, your brain will be available for more constructive use. Numbing it with the flickering phosphorous of someone else's vision of reality is not the way to improved family relationships, better communications, and personal conviction necessary to resume control of your life.

2. Begin an aggressive exercise program. Want more energy and endurance for the really important things in your life? Start exercising. Too tired at the end of the day? Exercise in the morning. Already late to the office? Get up earlier. Don't have the discipline? Hire a coach to make you accountable. Already exercising? Exercise even longer. The same way you make a muscle stronger is the same way you make yourself stronger, you stress it. While it seems like a contradiction in terms, using up energy will give you more. Lose those extra pounds and free up more personal power for your commitment to chiropractic.

3. Find a mentor. It hurts our egos but somewhere there's someone already doing what we want to do, and doing it better. Trying on a new success habit is easier when we watch someone else doing it. Find someone using your technique, experiencing the office volume you want, or getting the patient retention you want and spend a day or two with them. The loss of income will be quickly recovered by your renewed assurance and confidence when you return. Procedures or ideas holding you back that you thought were impossible to abandon become easier to dismiss when you see someone else "breaking the rules." Admit that you don't have all the answers. Realize no one has a corner on the truth. Not even your mentor!

4. Begin public speaking. Whip this one and nothing can hold you back. Practice this acquired skill with others similarly inclined. Get to a Toastmasters group as soon as possible. Being able to organize your thoughts, think on your feet, and share your point of view will improve every aspect of your life. The one thing that consistently separates successful offices from those less effective, is the ability to communicate. Risking your doctorly image and exposing yourself to an audience will pay off in ways you can't fathom.

These are just four simple suggestions. If they made you uncomfortable or seemed unrealistic; if you're almost sure you won't do any of them, please stop complaining. If it takes peer pressure to motivate you, then tell others you intend to start doing this or that. If it takes some other incentive to motivate you, reward yourself with some little luxury or indulgence as you adopt these new habits. If you need a gun to your temple to prompt a change, do nothing now. However, realize you are relinquishing control of your life and your future if you lack discipline. Because you can never be sure who will be holding the gun.

In the same way that buying a diet book (and even reading it) will not slim you down, simply reading these suggestions won't result in a better practice. Simply knowing it won't do. You must act. Your practice will improve only because *you* improve. Your practice will grow only because *you* grow. And your practice will be all that it can be when *you* become all that you can be. ■

HELPING
PATIENTS
CHANGE

As a writer and lecturer I'm fascinated by the challenge of personal change. Intuitively we all know that change is inevitable. We know the only thing we can count on is change. Yet, changing our habits or procedures or even our outlook on life is one of the most difficult things to do. We are all guilty of taking the path of least resistance—and wondering why we get the same results and the same frustrations. If making personal change is difficult, imagine the added challenge of helping facilitate change in others!

As I've shared my ideas with doctors and staff, conducted consultations, and spoken with hundreds of patients in focus group settings, I've developed a model of how people change. This model has been helpful in reframing my own reality and has allowed personal growth and satisfaction beyond my wildest imagination. Perhaps it will help you too.

1. Problem. Identifying the problem, articulating the situation I'm unhappy with, or clearly labeling what it is I want is the first step. This may be the most important aspect of all. It is important to diagnose the cause, otherwise the resulting symptom chasing disguises the problem and it further eludes me. Obviously being able to see the trees in the context of the forest is important. If I can't see enough context to allow me to identify the cause, I allow this ambiguity to exist and move to the next step anyway. The key point here is that if you're comfortable with the status quo and don't see a problem, don't expect change. Your world is apparently in a homeostatic balance and action is not required.

2. Information. The next thing I do is collect data and look for patterns. It is often during this information-gathering stage that the true cause emerges. This is when the ability to ask questions, of yourself and others, is so important. If your problem isn't to find the unified theory of the universe, someone, somewhere probably has information or an opinion that could help. Ask open-ended questions. Questions that can't be answered with a yes or a no. "What do you think about..." or "What's been you're experience when..." or "What do you do when..." Open ended questions are fluid and prevent dogma or preconceived notions block your exploration. If the cause doesn't reveal itself—keep looking.

3. Visualization. The writer in *Proverbs* was correct when observing that "Without vision the people perish." At this stage I start visualizing possible outcomes of implementing various possible solutions. The key is to be willing to reject the first possible solution. The best idea or most elegant approach doesn't always arrive first. Sometimes I find it helpful to imagine what it would take to create the exact opposite effect that I want and then work backwards from there. Regardless, it is important to "see" the outcome in your mind's eye. Like chess grand masters who play eight and 10 moves ahead, it is critical to play out possible solutions in advance. If you cannot "see" the solution or change in place, it is unlikely to ever happen.

4. Imbalance. This is the most difficult to describe, yet it is the most essential if true change is going to occur. If the visualization process does not create a great enough difference from the status quo to be compelling for action, don't expect change in behavior. The perceived improvement in esteem, efficiency, or other forms of tangible or intangible reward must be great enough to compel you to action. You must believe there will be an adequate gain or return on your investment. Without this imbalance between the status quo and the possibility of your vision, change is unlikely. Like deep ruts on a dirt road, setting a new course requires strength to abandon a sure thing. This is why little changes and minor modifications are more evident in our lives than the violent rejections of the status quo.

5. Affirmation. Because we live in a culture of instant gratification, some type of almost immediate positive feedback is essential to reinforce the change as we are making it. The element of time in the equation of change is often overlooked or we use the wrong scale. How many times have we instituted a new procedure only to abandon it before giving it enough time to actually work? To sustain the unrewarded effort during the early stages of change it is often helpful to review the images conjured up during the Visualization process. In this way you create your own feedback even if it doesn't reflect your current reality. This is easiest to do when the vision is most congruent with your key values, purpose, or mission in life—and most difficult to continue when our motives for change are self-serving or endanger or limit others. During this stage it is helpful to take small steps toward your intended results. If these small incursions into uncharted territory are met with a pleasant response, continue. If not, regroup.

6. Results. This is the change we wanted in the first place. If we give ourselves the freedom to adapt to the process along the way, the final results may be different than our original vision, however it may be easier to sustain. If our changed behavior exacts too high a toll on our resources (time, money, energy, status, etc.) then the results (changed behavior or attitude) don't last. Only if this new reality serves our needs, do we allow it to continue and become a habit. Otherwise the search starts over again.

This model can be helpful in explaining patient compliance, referrals, willingness to embrace maintenance care, and countless other patient behaviors.

Review this six-step process in the context of moving a patient from a sickness/medical model of health (treat the symptoms) to a wellness model of health and ultimately adopting a "chiropractic lifestyle." Briefly, here are the challenges facing you as a change agent:

1. Problem. The problem that prompts most patients to seek your office is an ache or a pain they think or hope you can help with. But the real problem is how to get a patient to think "cause" instead of "effect" and to understand their problem has been around longer than last week when they bent over and heard a popping sound.

2. Information. This is where patient education plays such an important role. If effective change is to occur, patients must understand the full nature and severity of their current condition and the behavior or health attitudes that led to their current situation.

3. Visualization. If patients can't "see what you mean" there is little hope that they will follow your recommendations. Your mission is to find out if the patient is motivated by moving "towards" something (wellness, restful sleep, better golf game) or by moving "away" from something (pain, degeneration, etc.) Speed the healing process by encouraging patients to visualize the outcome they want.

4. Imbalance. If improving and maintaining their health is not enough of a priority, as is the case with many patients, this step is the most challenging. If your usual patient education efforts do not create enough of an imbalance between what is and what could be, associate continued chiropractic care with something they're likely to value more. If you think you can help a new patient, ask them, "What do you hope to do better or enjoy more, when you regain your health?" Refer to this key value during subsequent visits as they receive care.

5. Affirmation. Short of a one visit miracle cure, relief care takes time. This early stage of care requires constant feedback and encouragement. Patients who have been taught to feel the instant relief from pain medication may lose patience with chiropractic unless your patient education helps change their expectations and adequate affirmation is offered along the way.

6. Results. If your patients don't get the results you had in mind, it simply means you weren't effective in helping them visualize the role of chiropractic in their health, and creating enough of an imbalance from their previous behavior to motivate them to make significant change. Perhaps your proposed change exacts too high a toll on their pocketbook or time away from their family after a long day at the office.

Changing the way patients think about their health and the value they place on themselves is one of the key responsibilities of doctors and staff members. For most patients, providing them with pain relief is a "no-brainer." The real challenge is not in the improvement of their spinal biomechanics, it is in helping patients change. ■

CONTROL AND
MANAGEMENT

We can only control that which is less powerful than ourselves. Controlling dogs, children, staff members, and small electrical appliances is relatively easy. Our experience, intellect, size, strength, or financial power make it easy for us to take control and guide our relationships in the way we wish. This sense of power and control can be quite addictive.

Patients who enter your office in severe pain are certainly less powerful than you. This makes it relatively easy to control patients during the early stages of their care. When you ask patients to complete four pages of admitting paperwork, they do. When you tell patients to stand in front of the X-ray bucky, they do. When you tell patients to apply some ice, they usually do. Because of their symptomatic condition they are compliant and seem to willingly obey your every command. Because of your clinical experience and a true desire to help, you direct patients in a care program that is in their best interests.

The consent to direct and control patients' behavior is a perishable commodity. As their symptoms disappear and they become more powerful, the patients' own "internal doctors" take over, modifying your suggestions; even openly disagreeing with your recommendations. Compliance suffers. Clearly, the patient management techniques that work during the initial stages of care aren't as effective when patients regain their health (and power).

I know a practice that was recently sold. The previous doctor was proud of his mix of patients and had attracted many families and influential white collar workers. In fact, his patients were a lot like him, reflecting his confidence, optimism, and sophistication. As when many practices are sold, the demographics of this office began to change. After the transition period when both doctors were in the office, patient volume began to drop off and then level out. The most striking thing about this sale and transition was what I observed a year later. Instead of a vibrant office of highly-educated professionals seeking wellness care, the practice had become filled with personal injury and blue collar worker's compensation cases. Apparently the new doctor was uncomfortable working with patients who were his peers and found it easier to control those who were less demanding and often less discerning.

In the same way we can feel underdressed in an upscale restaurant, doctors often inadvertently implement procedures or project an attitude or lack of confidence that makes certain patients feel unwelcome. A homeostatic balance is reached, based on the doctor's comfort level, self-esteem, social skills, personality, and energy level.

Where are the influencers of your community? The mayor, the city council, and business leaders? Everyone deserves access to chiropractic care, but the fact is, in all too many offices the doctor has unconsciously or purposely gone after the types of patients that are easiest to manage and control.

Same with staff. Some offices are blessed with independent, self-confident staff members who are free to speak their minds at staff meetings. They have a career attitude and have a sense of ownership in the practice. Other offices have people behind desks who are still looking for a clue as to who they are and why they're on this planet. They are easy to control, especially when they are kept in constant fear of losing their jobs if they make a mistake.

Which office is having more fun and making a greater impact on their community?

If you want to attract more influencers into your office and enjoy a staff that's pulling with you, you will need to recognize the difference between being a controlling authoritarian manager or a coaching facilitator and mentor.

The old school: The control and management school of thought believes that if given the chance people will goof off, make mistakes, and generally can't be trusted to do the right things. Those who ascribe to this Neanderthal way of thinking assume the burdensome task of orchestrating a patient's every move. Even in a day and age that has seen the socialism model crumble in Europe, there are still doctors who scare patients, badger patients for visits they don't understand they need, and make evening lectures mandatory.

The right to fail: If you've ever coached little league baseball you know the frustration (and joys) of coaching. The fundamental truth is that coaches cannot guarantee success, they can only teach the fundamental skills that it takes to win. This is why patient education is so important. You must empower patients with the information, lifestyle skills, and other resources they need to win. Remember though, it's their body, their spine, their health, and their future. Allow them the dignity to fail if they wish. They didn't appoint you den mother!

Set a good example: In a mentoring relationship based on mutual respect, a doctor must set a nonjudgmental example that a patient can find attractive. A doctor and staff must give patients something to shoot for. They must be living testimonials of the behavior they'd like their patients to adopt. That means physically, mentally, and socially. Your leadership role requires that you expand their vision.

Being liked versus being respected: This can be a most challenging aspect of leadership. All of us deeply desire to be accepted and liked. I don't know anyone who doesn't. The danger of this attitude is that it makes you as weak or weaker than those you are to lead. The best doctors challenge patients in a way that prompts them to want to do their best. Constant encouragement, open feedback, and frequent progress reports are important. Rarely do we do our best work in a vacuum. We all need constant affirmation that we're doing the right thing.

Willingness to delegate: It's certainly more expedient to just do it ourselves rather than explain how to do it to someone else. "In the time I could teach my staff I could do it myself!" wails a doctor in frustration on the phone. Doctors must delegate responsibilities to staff and patients. Chiropractic is participative in this regard. Patients need to keep up their side of the bargain for optimum results. This involvement enhances self-esteem, improves the healing process, and is the hallmark of self-reliance and trust necessary in long term relationships.

Nondefensive posture: Most of us learn best by experience. When you allow patients to fail by dropping out of care early, remind them that you will always be available should their problem return. Make sure they know you'll welcome them back without an "I-told-you-so." Help prevent them from going down the street to save face or giving up on chiropractic because they might be afraid to confront you a year or two later.

Control is a myth. The ambiguity that would result if the full reality of this notion were realized by most of us would cause panic and chaos. The fact that any patient returns after the first visit is a testimonial to your ability to lead and influence. Similarly, if patients drop out after seven visits because they feel better, it is a reflection of your communication skills and leadership ability. You can't have it both ways.

In the end, the only thing you can control is yourself. If you lack the discipline and courage needed to do the right thing, don't expect your patients to rise to the occasion. Patients are watching you. They're studying how you lead your life, your practice, your marriage, your staff, and your daily conduct. Start with the who you see in the mirror. ■

ADDICTED
TO POWER

When we use our power and influence to fashion the world around us, we are in a sense playing God. Part of the heady experience of running a business is in the fulfillment of a creation in our own image. This notion has been institutionalized in the countless rags to riches stories that surround the likes of Carnegie, Rockefeller, and other captains of industry in the early 1900s. Building an empire in which dutiful lieutenants stand at your beck and call to execute your every wish makes exciting drama. This sense of power and control is as addictive as any narcotic and perhaps more dangerous. It is especially enticing in the world of health care, surrounded by miracle cures and the proximity to the vital forces of life, death, and disease.

Some might call it "being doctorly" or simply assuming the symptoms of having once been put on a pedestal due to your education and social position. Yet it is this persona, this mask, that serves to separate and insulate you. Not just from possible failure, but from the "connectedness" patients so desperately want from their health care providers.

Abandoning this mask in favor of a more personal relationship with patients is difficult because this persona appears to assist in the control and management of patients. At least in the short term.

This is exhibited throughout the typical doctor/patient relationship in many chiropractic offices. Many of the compliance and new patient shortcomings can be traced to a lack of rapport and trust that is compromised by exploiting the powerful position you purposely or inadvertently find yourself in.

Telephone screening: Can patients actually talk to the doctor? In many offices the doctor is so afraid of confronting creditors or headrest paper salesmen that every phone call is carefully screened. Stop hiding. During your off-peak hours take some calls without screening. Really feeling bold? Answer the second line yourself! The worse that could happen from displaying this attractive quality of accessibility is you'll get tied up for a few minutes with a stock broker. "I'm sorry, but I'm not interested" can put a quick end to anyone's sales pitch. If not, putting the handset back on the phone is guaranteed to work! By taking a few calls you'll become more sensitive to the needs of your patients and get a better feel for how your office functions. This is the same exercise countless Fortune 500 executives experience by spending a day serving hamburgers, handling hotel guests' luggage, or taking airplane passengers' tickets. It's too easy to get isolated in the back room trudging between three adjusting rooms.

Reception room: Many doctors meet patients for the first time in a cramped consultation room. This is disorienting for patients who, after spending 12 minutes completing your admitting paperwork, are just now feeling comfortable with the reception area portion of your office. Being taken to still another part of this strange new place reminds patients they are powerless and are subject to someone else's agenda and protocol. Want to impress patients with your self-confidence and accessibility? Come out to the reception room, be introduced to the patient by a staff member, and lead them back to the consultation room yourself!

The examination: This is often when the doctor is most powerful, using esoteric tests and all-knowing "Hmmms" at just the right time to project a sense of thoughtful assessment and learned understanding. When doctors don't communicate what they're finding as they're finding it, it reminds patients that they're the patient and you're the doctor. If you enjoy this control and suspense to later exploit at your report of findings, please know that it's counterproductive. Oh, sure, patients can hardly wait to see their X-rays, but without foreshadowing your findings at your examination, you run the risk of numbing the patient with too much information. Gain greater understanding and respect for your recommendations by letting patients get a basic understanding of positive test results as they occur. Otherwise, the result is a patient who is resentful and selectively remembers only bits and pieces of your oral report.

X-ray procedures: While taking X-rays in many offices is a fore drawn conclusion, this is where the skirmishes of an intimidation game are frequently played out. Patients walk into your X-ray room with four basic concerns: privacy, necessity, safety, and cost. Since many patients lack the willingness to confront, especially when they are disadvantaged by discomfort, many doctors are lured into thinking these four issues don't even exist! Making the effort to anticipate, acknowledge, and volunteer relevant information about these often unspoken issues will pay huge dividends in less confrontation, better questions, and more cooperative patients. To simply push this or any other procedure down a patient's throat without explanation because, "This is how we do things around here" may put an immediate end to the objections, but it creates a climate of resentment and compliance through gritted teeth.

The report of findings: Besides avoiding the manipulative scare tactics which no longer work with the baby boom generation, the major flaw in many reports is the unwillingness to discuss financial matters with the patient. Too bad. Offices in which doctors help patients fully appreciate the relationship of their visit schedule, fees, and probable recovery time also have higher collections, better compliance, and, get this, more referrals. Is this reluctance because you secretly feel the $30 adjustment fee and the $320 Davis Series is overpriced? Is it because you get *your* care without any impact to your monthly budget? Or, is it because you live and breathe chiropractic 24 hours a day that you automatically think patients will too? If you think patients draw a distinction between optimum health care and their pocket books, you're kidding yourself. Health care costs money. And unless you can effectively communicate the cost/benefit ratio of following your recommendations, most patients won't. The fact is, many aren't.

Recall procedures: As patients vote with their feet and discontinue care when they are as powerful as you (symptom-free), the crowning touch of a power-based practice is deployed: the recall. With carefully scripted phone dialogue and an urgent, "the doctor has discovered something on your X-rays," the front desk assistant suddenly turns into Nurse Ratchet. Besides the fact that it's so distasteful that the staff member with the least amount of seniority is given this dirty little task, it's often done within earshot of patients in the reception room! Heavy-handed recall programs are the last gasp of a health care "dictator" and acknowledges a lack of patient education and loss of control. Plus, they only produce short-term results and sabotage a long-term relationship. Live by the sword. Die by the sword.

Besides the fact that using power and control strategies with patients and staff members is so gratifying to our egos, the real problem is it appears to work! Countless staff members are working at a fraction of their productivity because they are in fear of losing their jobs or unsure how well they are doing their jobs. Fear and intimidation produce staff members who lose their ability to make even the simplest decision, requiring constant direction from the boss. This feeds the supervisor's ego, further reinforcing the notion to think for everyone else in the office. The self-fulfilling prophecy that is created makes the boss even less likely to delegate and empower others. High staff turnover, constant use of sick leave, and tardiness are all symptoms of staff-related "power pathology." When exercised on patients the symptoms include low compliance, few referrals, and poor patient visit average.

That doesn't mean babying your patients, becoming their "friend," or striving to be liked by your patients is the solution either! You need to confront patients out of love. You need to present specific recommendations out of leadership. And you need to educate out of the responsibility that comes from knowing the truth. ■

GETTING
RESPECT

Research suggests that the information needed to replicate each of us is encoded on each genetic ribbon of our chromosomes. Embedded in each gene is the collected information of our species and our hereditary past. In our every muscle fiber is the history of tribal campfires and ritual. In every sinew the connectedness to nature lies dormant. We have become "civilized" and transcended the shaman, the cave paintings, and the wonder of the rising sun, the changing seasons, and the awareness of the miracle we call life.

Don't worry, your patients have too!

The separation of our educated mind and our "primitive" body has corrupted us. It has changed who we are. It has modified the environment. It has severely influenced our relationships. How else can you explain the destruction of the rain forests, the pollution of our rivers, and the carcinogenic chemicals we feed the animals that we eat, and the way we treat our elders?

We are the problem.

Most of us have surrounded ourselves with people who like us. Who are reluctant to criticize us. Who won't tell the emperor he or she isn't wearing any clothes. It works great. We pretend to be the boss, and they pretend to care. We pretend to be responsible and they pretend to like the status quo. We pretend we're making a difference, and they pretend to love their job.

Cozy, isn't it?

The "higher up" you get, the more serious the problem. Yet, even in medieval times the king recognized this, entertaining the joker to sanction dissent and to be the voice for the public; the little people. The joker or court jester was an important person in the royal court. His job was to question the status quo. To ask the "what if" questions. To poke fun. To jab. To force the royal court to look at issues of the day in a new way. We all need court jesters.

Yet, somehow we think we can maintain the status quo or protect our fragile self-esteem by isolating ourselves from the opinions of the people who depend on us (and we on them). We kid ourselves, thinking a strong-armed approach to staff relations will insure productivity. We think keeping staff members in a constant state of fear of losing their job will motivate them to be more conscientious. We think that saying "three times a week means three times a week and if you miss your appointment we expect you to make it up" will automatically result in optimal compliance. We think that just "doing a good job" will assure patient satisfaction and fulfillment.

Today, do-as-I-say doesn't work. Oh sure, for the generation born during the Depression, the authoritarian approach works pretty well. They tend to place the all-knowing doctor on a pedestal and look for direction and limits. Just try that with a 35-year old college educated baby boomer! It doesn't work. Maybe for a short time through clenched teeth, but it's not the tenacious kind of compliance that is bred from respect.

The question is, would you rather be respected or would you rather be liked? Think about it before you choose! There are significant ramifications to your choice.

Certainly it's easier to be liked than to be respected. Being liked means there's no need to confront a patient (spouse, child, etc.) and you can abandon any concerns about the future. Live for the moment. Decisions and directions given to others tend to be on the safe side, avoiding conflict at all costs. The path of least resistance is a very crowded road. It is a type of slavery, succumbing to the lowest common denominator. Like patients who don't necessarily want to be healthy, just pain free, doctors find themselves trapped in a practice which becomes repetitious and unfulfilling. Wanting to be liked short-changes the future.

On the other hand, if you'd rather be respected, practice takes on a whole new dimension! Granted, it takes high self-esteem, purpose, passion, vision, and creativity. Since you chose chiropractic, it's going to take some extra effort:

Patient education: Patients cannot respect something they don't understand. The tendency is to devalue, reject, or be afraid of something we don't understand. Think back to the patients you've helped but who resisted or ignored your patient education efforts. Sure, many probably left feeling better, but they have no idea what you really did. No understanding. No referrals. No respect. Without patient education it's like practicing in the dark—you know you're doing a great job, but no one else does.

Set high standards: Remember that important coach or high school teacher? He or she demanded your very best. Your excellence or achievement was the result of high standards. Oh, at the time we hated the extra work. But later, even we were impressed with our newly developed abilities! The teachers who let you coast, who didn't demand much from you, who allowed you to cheat yourself are not held with much respect in your memory today. If you want respect, set high standards for you and your patients. You'll notice that as you improve the appearance of your office, your letterhead, and the letters you send, that other aspects of your practice suddenly look ripe for improvement too. Pick an area and do it just a little better.

Know yourself: People who command respect from us have a deep understanding of themselves and their own shortcomings. They are not perfect, but we see them making the best of the moment. They are not complainers. They may get angry at injustice or inefficiency, however they have a sense of calmness and confidence we find intriguing. They do not lie to themselves. They are unafraid of criticism, in fact, they often invite it. Self-knowledge is required for the boldness and courage to exceed expectation and confront mediocrity. Lead an open life.

Long term vision: The people we respect are more interested in the future than the past. Most of us find it difficult to concentrate on the same idea for more than a few minutes. People we respect never stop. They have a boundless energy and a focus that allows them to see the world as it could be, and not be bound by the world as it is. Their ability to delay gratification and explore the long-term ramifications of a decision or an action is a mark of a true leader.

Allow others to fail: This is often the most difficult. When you respect others, you honor them by being non-judgmental. (This is where your eternal optimism comes in handy!) When we see others short-change their lives by the decisions they make, it's only natural to want to intervene. Done improperly this intervention backfires. Be sure you explain the choices and the probable outcomes of each choice, and then let the patient decide. In the long run it pays off. If they discontinue care prematurely, their problem is likely to return. When it does, if they respect you, they'll return to your office and you'll get another chance. If they respect you.

You're it. The problem in most offices isn't procedures, or technique, or which college you graduated from, or whether you were the oldest son or the youngest daughter. It's you. It's easy to place the blame elsewhere, after all, there are so many culprits: the media, the insurance companies, the staff, the town, the weather, the patients...

It's you. While few people will tell you, if you want your patients to respect you, you have to start by respecting yourself. ■

DECIDING TO DECIDE

After six or eight years of practice the results are almost a cliché. The staff turns over about every two years or so. Patient volume is comfortable, but not newsworthy. Compliance is satisfactory if the patient has insurance. It's a nice little practice. Family is doing fine. Nice cars.

Ho-hum.

The excitement is gone. The idealistic "I'm-going-to-change-the-world-through-chiropractic" has atrophied. The reason for getting into chiropractic in the first place has been forgotten. Now, it's a living. Your practice has become comfortable. Maybe too comfortable.

The insurance industry tamed your passion nicely.

What grabs your attention now are the legislature's attempt to change the worker's compensation coverage. Self-preservation rekindles the spirit when the state considers capping personal injury awards. The pulse quickens when your patient's insurance agent lies that their automobile insurance doesn't cover chiropractic.

Funny what it takes to get our attention. Start tinkering with our finances and suddenly there's a hormonal imbalance and we're ready to fight.

But usually it's more talk than action. All too often state associations and chiropractic societies have to beg for money. At meetings when the hat is passed, the hallways and bathrooms are suddenly full. Has chiropractic become too easy?

Looked through any of profession's periodicals recently? It's enough to cause vertebral subluxations! The ads, the claims, and the promises of million dollar practices clutter virtually every page. Every "I'm-not-like-all-the-other-practice-management-firms" ad reduces chiropractic to a financial procedure. Every editorial whines about the RAND study or the *20/20* story or the Dear Abby column. "It's unfair," someone whimpers. "They put us in a box," someone else bemoans.

This is what chiropractic has been reduced to?

For a profession that claims to be interested in "cause" and not "symptoms", there sure is a lot of symptom chasing in the profession's periodicals! When the red headline proclaims, "I'll show you how to get more new patients than you'll ever need," that's treating symptoms. Why do most practices have a voracious appetite for new patients? Why don't patients remain for wellness care? Why don't current patients refer others to your office? Why can't patients afford care in your office? Why aren't there more children and families in your practice? How come your patients can't adequately describe to others what you do?

When you get real answers to questions like these, you'll more likely stop "practicing medicine" on your practice and start looking at cause. Correct the cause and the symptoms take care of themselves. Who wants to bite the bullet and wrestle with the true cause of a less-than-optimum practice?

Even as a nation we resist the pain and delayed gratification of looking for cause. We (and our elected officials) refuse to look our bazillion dollar deficit squarely in the face. We are in denial. To get re-elected no one mentions the elephant sleeping in the living room. Every two, four, and six years the names change, but nothing really changes. Except things get worse.

The management boys have perfected this dance by looking to financial statistics or new patient volumes as an easy judge of the health of a practice. If that type of shorthand only worked! Few management organizations have the courage to tell the truth. Because if they did, the doctors might not reup at the end of their contract. And so it goes. What could be a dynamic opportunity for personal and professional growth turns into a pep rally and a "things-are-okay-at-our-office" form of group denial. Too bad.

What are you going to do after you've heard all the Zig Ziglars of chiropractic and nothing really changes in your life and your practice? What are you going to do with another "this-will-change-your-life" set of audio tapes? How many more manuals do you need? How many more hours do you need to sit on those uncomfortable hotel chairs at seminars? What's it going to take to finally realize, that like each of our inborn potentials to heal ourselves, personal and practice growth is an inside job? When are you going to recognize that practice solutions, like health solutions, don't come from the outside?

You're it!

A new narrative to extract more money from insurance companies won't correct the cause. A new seminar promising a million dollar practice won't correct the cause. A new video, a new audio, a new this, or a revolutionary that, won't correct the cause. Only you can correct the cause. And it starts in the deciding. You must decide to confront the sometimes ugly and the sometimes embarrassing truth about you.

For many, this is a difficult decision. Some will wait until circumstances force the required change. Others will prolong the decision to the very last minute. Others will endure what they call their lives, from the cradle to the grave, without ever making the decision. Many will prefer to avoid the introspection required to confront their own lies. (Remember, the truth sets you free. Every time!)

Decide.

Careful! The ramifications of deciding are serious. Deciding will prompt changes. The people around you don't want you to change! It challenges their belief structure. It may cost you a friendship. It may cost you a lifestyle. It will cost. For some, this cost will prevent the personal and professional liberation necessary to have a great life and a great practice.

Decide.

Decide what you want. Decide what you need. Decide who you are. Decide what you want on your tombstone. Decide your purpose for being in chiropractic. Decide to get real and confront that dirty secret or that debilitating fear of yours. Decide to be an example of a "get real" life.

157

If these types of issues were being tackled at practice management seminars there would be little need for more than a once a year get-together to celebrate everyone's success. No reups. No new forms. No rah-rah. No corny jokes. No bragging. Once you know who you are and decide to live an open life, answers to questions about what forms to use and how to get new patients are embarrassingly obvious.

This isn't intended to be a "cookbook" for how to decide, but here are some observations that I've noticed in those I've met, who seem to make decisions effortlessly:

Purpose: It all starts here. If you don't know why you've been put on this planet, you're destined to wander aimlessly without making a real impact.

Values: If you're having a hard time deciding, you're probably not in touch with your own personal value system. How do you conduct yourself when no one is watching? What would you die for? What are your limits? What are your standards?

Outcome: What do you want? What measurable result or impact do you want to accomplish because of being in practice? Until you visualize (and that's important), the outcome you want, you are merely surviving.

Find a mentor: Even the president and the pope have advisors. Are you spending time with people who have the values and outcomes you want? Stop whining and commiserating with the little people. Find someone who will tell you the truth and push you to new limits.

High energy: Deciding can be hard work. It takes energy. Stop watching television and reading the newspaper. De-media your life. Start exercising. Get adjusted more regularly. Eat better food. Walk 30% faster.

Faith: You must believe in a power higher than yourself. Not as a crutch but as a benchmark for your spiritual growth. Seek out others that believe the same way you do. Worship. Get involved.

Notice that none of these aspects have anything directly to do with money. Instead of looking for the best tax-free municipal bonds, it means investing in yourself. You spend so much time and energy serving others and caring for your patients (even taking the disrespectful ones home with you at night), that it's time to invest in yourself. Remember, it's an inside job.

A successful life or a successful practice is a symptom. It is the result of many things. Until you are in touch with the cause of these attractive symptoms, satisfaction and personal growth will forever elude you. Before you become cynical or think chiropractic "did it to you" decide to take back your life. Decide to be selfish just long enough to find out who you really are. The first step is simply to decide to decide. The world will be a better place because of it. ■

DEAR
GRADUATE

This year thousands of new chiropractors will graduate and enter the work force in North America. Armed with the knowledge necessary to pass the national examination and the particular idiosyncratic obstacles of a state licensing board, these new doctors will discover that their education has just begun. The curriculum at most chiropractic colleges rarely provides sufficient direction necessary to exchange these valuable healing skills with patients in a win/win relationship.

A lot has changed since most of these students embarked on their chiropractic training four years ago:

1. The insurance environment has changed. Today $100 deductibles are merely a fond memory. Nowadays, fewer patients even have chiropractic coverage in their health insurance, are members of HMOs lacking chiropractic coverage, or have deductibles that match a typical case average!

2. There is more competition. Time was when a new graduate could begin practice in a small town and be the only chiropractor for miles around. Today there's a chiropractic office next to every shopping mall, yogurt stand, and convenience store. Differentiating their office from the chiropractor down the street is a challenge few doctors have had to face in the past.

3. The economy has changed. Lying to one's self, denying reality with a "positive mental attitude", or "deciding not to participate in the recession" ignores the fact that unemployment is up, credit card balances are being paid down, and confidence about the future is shaky. People are increasingly careful about their purchases—especially chiropractic because "once you start you have to go for the rest of your life."

These are significant changes that challenge status quo approaches for launching a new practice. No longer is it enough to simply locate a new office at a location suggested by a high traffic count. There's probably already a chiropractic office there, plus, it may not be in an area of town where the types of patients you'd especially enjoy serving live or work.

If I had just graduated, passed the state boards, and was ready to open my own practice, here are some of the things I'd do to prime the pump and get things rolling:

1. Develop my mission statement. It sounds so unglamorous and low tech that most graduates won't do it, but it's the most important thing you can do. Without articulating on paper the "what you want to do," "the who you want to do it with," "the how you're going to do it", and "the measurable result for having done it" you're in for a lot of frustration and unfulfilled pipe dreams. Brainstorm these components and fashion a short paragraph of three or four sentences that can serve as a benchmark for the first several years of practice. Your purpose can change as you mature, but you need a launching pad to get started.

2. Identify your ideal patient. Again, it sounds so unromantic at a time when you want to get your hands on some patients and see the power of chiropractic work, but if you don't, it's easy to wake up several years later, trapped in a practice you don't even like. I've talked to doctors who actually resent their patients! I bet you treat patients you especially enjoy serving better, than those whose poor hygiene or negative attitudes causes you to dislike them.

3. Become an associate. I know what you're thinking. You've got the money and the ambition to start off immediately on your own, but I wouldn't. The temptation to put school behind you and prove to the world that everyone else is wrong can be pretty compelling. But I'd want to get some experience in the real world before marching off to my own drummer. Sure, associate relationships are often win/lose, but take the slave wages and use it to perfect your technique, see how a real office functions, and build the tableside manners necessary to have a successful practice of your own.

4. Take a vacation. It's not what you're thinking! Find out the names of doctors who have a big vision for chiropractic, use a similar technique, and share your value system. Then take a trip. Make arrangements with several of these doctors in an area a day or two away by car, and take a tour. Go on rounds with the doctor. Ask questions in the hallway between patients. Buy the doctor a meal. Pick his or her brain. But most of all, soak up the headspace and the systems the doctor is using that allows the practice to make such an impact in their community. You might want to do things differently, but at least your brain will be enlarged by the experience.

5. Use direct mail. Shave off the facial hair, remove the ear ring, get your hair styled, and put on your best professional clothing. Then get a great photo of yourself taken. Contract with a graphic designer (use the yellow pages) and have them use this photo in a simple direct mail piece. Besides your photo include 1) a statement introducing yourself and your background, 2) some brief copy that overcomes some of the misconceptions about chiropractic and why you're different, 3) explain your availability by phone during a certain time on a certain day of the week to answer any type of health question anonymously over the phone with no obligation, and 4) a call to action to find out what the "latest state-of-the-art chiropractic is all about." Mail it to a 3-5 mile radius of your new office.

6. Start outside speaking. Deny it if you want, work around it if you have to, but your ability to speak at civic groups, senior citizen luncheon programs, and other community get togethers is one of the best and least expensive exposures for chiropractic and you. Plant seeds that may take days, weeks, months, or years to bear fruit. The key is to get out of your "box" and share what you do with complete strangers. Overcoming the fear of public speaking will make the fear of practice failure seem like small potatoes!

7. Conduct office tours. Make sure that everyone who even pokes their head into your office gets a tour and an explanation of chiropractic. Before you give the UPS delivery person the signature they want, drag them around your office and give a three-minute explanation of chiropractic. Same with the phone installation person, the water delivery person, the cleaning people, and the copy machine salesperson. Just asking for salespeople to come to your office for bids on your telephone system, copy machine needs, letterhead and business card printing, and liability insurance could keep you busy with countless opportunities to explain chiropractic to potential patients!

8. Send congratulation letters or postcards. Spend time each day clipping articles in the local newspaper announcing births, achievements in slow pitch softball league, promotions, and other accomplishments. Use the city directory at the library during your lunch hour to find addresses. Mail these "famous" people a copy of the article. Include a blurb about yourself and the "success" you offer patients or the "promotion" of good health you offer, or the "winning" ways you have with many types of health problems. Don't over do it—just a line or two. Your mission is simply a method of getting your name out in a classy way that avoids a hard sell.

Between your office tours, newspaper clipping, and telephone consultations you should be pretty busy. If you're not exhausted at the end of the day, here are some things to consider doing after hours while you're chomping at the bit for tomorrow to come:

9. Work out. It sounds strange but you need to be in shape to handle the stress and pressure. The only way to do that is to be in tip top physical condition. Plan to give yourself 20 to 30 minutes of vigorous physical exercise every day. Increase your lung capacity and the health of your cardiovascular system. Get ready to handle the demand for your unique and highly-effective approach to health care.

10. Rent some movies. It's time for inspiration! Go out and rent some of the early *Rocky* movies. Search out films that show ordinary people overcoming great obstacles to right a wrong or carry the banner of truth and justice forward. When I need a kick in the pants I rent *Tucker* and *Field of Dreams*. They always get me back on track.

11. Read non-chiropractic books. Since you've got chiropractic figured out now, the remaining uncharted territory is how to think like a successful small business person. Read some books that explain the relationship between customers and service providers. My favorites are *The E-Myth* by Michael Gerber, *How to Win Customers and Keep Them*

For Life by Michael LeBoeuf, Ph.D., *Customers For Life* by Carl Sewell, *Marketing Without Advertising* by Michael Phillips and Salli Rasberry, and *Positively Outrageous Service* by T. Scott Gross.

Maybe you don't feel comfortable with all of these ideas, but somewhere here you should feel empowered to go forth with confidence, knowing thousands of chiropractors go before you, proving it's possible. I'm sure there are many other ideas, but these should get you started and still allow you to respect yourself in the morning. Congratulations and good luck! ∎

BASEBALL AND COMMITMENT

I was confiding my frustration with an associate the other day, complaining that many of my projects weren't getting off the ground or enjoying the success I thought they should. His advice was a harpoon of truth that not only got me out of feeling sorry for myself, but the techniques he revealed to renew my commitment may be helpful to you.

"It's a question of commitment," he said over his breakfast meeting pancakes in a way that suggested how obvious the solution was to him.

"Commitment?" I volunteered, not recognizing the brilliance of his insight. "Why is it always so hard to self-diagnose?" I asked myself.

"Sure, you're going through what I did, trying this, dabbling in that, launching projects and waiting for the thunderous applause to help you make up your mind as to which project or idea to fully invest your life spirit in."

That hurt. But secretly I knew he was right. While I had been patting myself on the back for all my recent output, it hadn't given me the fulfillment I desired.

"What do you mean, life spirit?" I asked coyly giving me time to search for something less personal to blame.

"Life spirit, 100%, 'the juice,' going for it; passion. Investing every-thing you've got in the belief you've got a winner. You can't hold anything back. Ever been bankrupt?" he asked, seemingly changing the subject.

"No," I answered proudly.

"Too bad. We probably wouldn't be having this discussion if you'd ever gone through bankruptcy," he said. "If you had, you'd be dangerous because with your ideas, your skills, and ability to communicate them, you wouldn't fear failure."

I took another bite of my waffle, savoring the food and the food for thought as my mind went racing. He was right. I had been conditioned to be "right." Our culture taught me to be right. The more right answers on a test in school, the better you were. Too many wrong answers and you failed. To avoid failure you had to be right over 50% of the time. Yet, using the same scale you'd be reading this by candlelight because Edison would never have made the hundreds of tries (and failures) needed to find the right material for a light bulb filament.

Yes, I was afraid of failure. I'd been hedging my bet so I'd have an out; a way of saving face. By keeping my distance from my project and not giving it 100% I could always deny my relationship to my project, idea, or creative offspring. If you judged my idea you were judging me. Yet, if I distanced myself from my creations (your practice, your volume, your patient visit average, post X-ray changes, etc.) I could protect my fragile ego.

To compensate, I became a victim of over achievement. I started creating more and more and doing more and more while diluting my impact. Statistically things looked good, but I missed the satisfaction that comes from 100% commitment.

"Few people hit home runs every time at bat and few people come up with ideas that take off without effort or total commitment," he said.

"Yeah, I've heard the one about Babe Ruth striking out all those times," I quickly volunteered, hoping to keep the discussion on a more practical level.

Instead of Ruth, he told me about Ted Williams, the only major league baseball player with a lifetime batting average of .400. Apparently he had 10/20 vision; better than most people. It is thought his enhanced vision helped him to see the ball more clearly and judge whether a pitch was within the strike zone. Williams was known for not swinging at pitches outside the strike zone. In a rare interview, Williams was asked why. "You'd probably still hit a lot of them and have an even higher batting average," the sports writer conjectured.

"But then I'd never know where to draw the line," answered Williams.

My mind was racing. Apparently commitment is the result of knowing where to draw the line. If you've clearly identified your values, you can set absolute standards for your conduct and improve your ability to make the right decision during moments of stress or conflict. This focus (10/20) comes from having a clearly identified value system. Gone is the opportunity chasing and the fragmentation that is all too often the symptoms of a lack of commitment.

"I think you've made an accurate observation," I volunteered slowly, feeling more lost and dejected with each passing moment. It was of little consolation that I was experiencing the very normal state of depression that signals the personal growth before an important breakthrough. "So what's the next step," I asked, already knowing the answer.

"What do you want? Why do you want to do it? How do you want to do it? With whom do you want to do it? What result do you want for having done it?" he asked, parroting off the same five components of a statement of purpose I used to teach.

Suddenly I heard myself make the same argument I had heard from doctors at seminars, "Yeah, but I don't need philosophy, I need to know what to do right now." Even my voice was taking on the tinge of desperation I had heard so frequently in private, one-on-one consultations.

Recognizing there weren't any shortcuts, I began the process of inspecting my statement of purpose. And I discovered something about myself that I had diagnosed in a doctor just weeks earlier: I'm a poor delegator. Without delegating to employees to carry out portions of my vision, I am limited by what I can do personally. Sound familiar?

As he finished his pancakes in silence and I my waffles, I was deep in thought. I was comforted by the friendship that didn't demand filling the air with conversation.

"So you think it's just a matter of commitment?" I volunteered distantly. "Yup."

"And if I get committed, success, and recognition will follow?"

"Right."

"So, what's the first step?"

"Act as if you already have it," he said cleaning the last of the maple syrup off his plate.

"Pretend? Isn't that a lot like lying?"

"No, it's visualizing the outcome you want. It's modeling the desirable behavior you see in someone else that you'd like to have in yourself. It's related to identifying your purpose. It's a form of goal setting."

"How do I act like I'm already committed?" I asked growing interested in the process as much as the outcome.

"Describe to me some of the characteristics of a committed person. Give me the names of some of the people you recognize as being committed."

"Ralph Nader. Mother Teresa. Jack Kemp. Frank Lloyd Wright. William F. Buckley."

"Good. What are some of the characteristics of the people you named?"

"Well, they all seem to have a passion about them," I volunteered.

"What else?"

"They each seem attached to some type of cause," I said thinking out loud. "They have a point of view."

"And?"

"I suppose some people viewed them as different. Even disagree with them."

"Bingo," he said. "Imagine the courage of an Edison who keeps trying. Or the confrontation that results from a woman like Mother Teresa who does the kinds of things all of us should be doing. Or the self-confidence of a Nader who keeps pushing up against the largest corporations."

It is said the truly happy people are people who are bothered. They have a cause. The meaning they derive from life is attached to something larger than what they can accomplish by themselves, for themselves. Only until you are bothered by something can you have the commitment necessary for success.

What's bothering you? ■

KILLING
SNAKES

I'm not particularly fond of snakes. There's something about their scaly appearance and deceptive nature that bothers me. They hide (a snake in the grass). They slither on their bellies. They are sneaky. They are deceptive. They can be a hidden threat.

Ever killed a snake? On several levels there is something primitive about the act. If you've ever killed a rattlesnake you know what I mean. It usually takes but one carefully positioned stroke, when using a shovel. Yet no one I know stops at this modest commitment of energy. No, when you kill a snake you go beyond the necessary. In an unexplainable and needless use of force, every fiber of your body is focused on the destruction of this largely helpful and innocent reptile.

Our family has a saying that describes this phenomena when applied to anything from cleaning the house to washing the car. "He's going at _____ like killing snakes." Killing snakes is a metaphor we use to describe anyone's total commitment in getting something done. Sometimes it means someone is going overboard and is being just a bit overzealous in their efforts.

It isn't a pretty metaphor, but it is powerful.

Whether you're a front desk C.A., choreographing a spectacular Monday evening rush hour, or a doctor writing a report, I hope you're doing it with "killing snakes" intensity. I believe it was the business consultant Tom Peters who said, "Excellence is never the result of moderation." When you inventory people you know who are enjoying life, a common denominator is an intense sense of passion in their work (or play) that is infectious. Think of the preachers, doctors, salespersons, and others who have attained high levels of success and recognition. What they share, regardless of vocation, is singleness of purpose. Ironically, away from the pulpit, or the patient, or the sales prospect, these individuals are often perceived as one dimensional and not having fun. So committed and focused, to outsiders they are often seen as humorless taskmasters. Don't be fooled. The real "juice" in living comes with total, 100% commitment. They're having fun—I can guarantee it.

Don't confuse constant opportunity chasing or simply being busy with a killing snakes attitude! There's much more to it. Being relentlessly busy and having your attention distracted from the latest emergency leads to burnout. What I'm talking about is the fulfillment that comes from the joyous and total immersion in a project or the subject at hand. Time stands still, yet when you finally are prompted to look at a clock, hours have passed. There is a connectedness in the moment.

If you want to start "killing snakes" in your office and unleash the power of 100% commitment, here are some tips from an especially experienced snake killer I know:

Awareness: It sounds so obvious, but first you have to see the snake. Yet you'd be surprised how many people can't see real or potential snakes. Their feedback loops and lack of sensitivity make it difficult for them to see opportunities for service. They neglect to recognize calls for help or "read the trail" of our times and anticipate the future. It requires openness. Those suffering from bigotry or prejudice of any kind need not apply. If you like the status quo, you're too comfortable. The truly happy people I've met are bothered about something. You first need a pet peeve or special project to get completely committed. In chiropractic this could take on the interest in building more of a cash practice, becoming an accomplished public speaker for chiropractic in your community, patient education techniques, developing the pediatrics aspect of your practice, or becoming an expert in some area of the profession. Analyze the trends you're seeing in your practice. Look for opportunities.

Purpose: Each of us is here for a purpose. Have you discovered yours yet? No snakes will fear for their lives until you do! This is much more than goal setting—which is critical, too. Your "purpose" often emerges when your skills and interests are in sufficient alignment so your vocation and avocation are one and the same. Snakes laugh at doctors who do things in their offices that should be delegated to others. Buying office supplies? Tracking X-ray film inventory? Cleaning the bathroom? Stay on purpose! Just because you can file X-rays, doesn't mean you should. When you're in touch with your purpose the decisions to ignore, postpone, or delegate responsibilities in your office are easier. Become a better steward of your skills and training.

Proper Tools: Killing snakes with your bare hands is not recommended. The proper tools make the job easier and faster. Sometimes the proper tool is simply a brain that is unencumbered by a limiting attitude, avoiding negative people, or constantly reminding yourself of your vision for the future. Do you have the resources in your office to get the job done? Do you have the horsepower? Is your staff similarly committed or are they just passing through on their way to something else? What's the condition of your adjusting table? Does the copy machine have the features your staff needs? Do you have enough phone lines? Do you have a mechanism to consistently educate your patients? How are your office systems functioning? When mistakes occur, do you blame people or systems (or the lack of systems)? The right tools in the hands of a craftsman is a very valuable thing.

Plan: Without a plan, valuable time and energy is wasted, and this bothers snake killers, who favor efficiency. While it looks to the bystander that snake killers have boundless energy, the best snake killers quickly lose interest when the return on their "energy investment" isn't sufficiently great enough. Obviously they have well-refined procedures and policy manuals. But don't be fooled by the obviousness of these tangible artifacts! They know where they're going and they have a plan to get them there. But any good snake killer worth his or her salt is open to new possibilities. They plan for unforeseen contingencies. They always know what to do if "the ball is thrown to them." So while they have a plan, they trust themselves enough to make revisions and exploit fortuitous windfalls.

Act: This is where amateur snake killers are revealed. Snake killers are doers. Merely planning, visualizing, or having a positive mental attitude won't do. Snake killers go boldly without reservation. They are champions of new ideas and sticklers for details. They willingly risk making a mistake or appearing foolish. Probably because they are caught up enjoying the moment, they don't worry what others think. Yet, because they believe in themselves and have properly laid the ground-work, they rarely fail. This is where their 100% commitment and total presence in the moment are so helpful—they get the job done! Novice snake killers who become preoccupied with snake bites or other distract-ing fears often find these ruminations become self-fulfilling prophecies. Experienced snake killers focus on the outcome and have a clear picture of the goal posts. They are not self-conscious. When you're killing snakes, form is not important—results are.

Clean up: Whenever you kill snakes there is always a mess. So it is advisable to take steps to restore order and take inventory of the situation. This willingness to conduct a post-mortem is a valuable feedback device that completes the cycle, going back to the awareness needed for improved snake killing in the future. After you clean up, celebrate. Beginner snake killers often overlook this important aspect. Instead of the countless successes, too many would-be snake killers take home the failures, remember the lost opportunities, or spend staff meetings re-counting the "ones that got away." Acknowledge disappointments and then move on. Be sure to smell the roses and bask in the glow of your accomplishment.

Everyone has a pet project, that when mentioned, causes a sparkle in their eyes or an infectious smile. Mihaly Csikszentmihalyi in his book, *Flow, The Psychology of Optimum Experience*, calls this feeling "flow." "In the flow," and "go with the flow" are two phrases that reveal the attitude of someone truly in the moment. When you're killing snakes you are totally "in the flow" and things happen without forcing them. There is efficiency and economy of movement. There is directness with finesse. There is elegance.

Killed any snakes lately? ■

IT'S YOUR
FAULT

The real tension in consulting work, whether you're a doctor, lawyer, management expert, or interior decorator is that quite often most people don't want to change. The status quo, as uncomfortable as it may be, is at least predictable. Most of us choose the defined over the potential; the "is" over the "what could be."

Someone once described a consultant as someone who uses your watch to tell you what time it is. Other definitions less complimentary exist too. However, this natural temptation to cling to the present order of things, wishing things were different, but feeling secure in the familiar, is what tests the mettle of the best consultants. Ironically, to call a consultant one must first admit that he or she has a problem, which is another stumbling block consultants must face: no one wants to admit they have a problem! If there isn't a problem, why is a consultant needed? So, the consultant's first responsibility is to assure the client that everything is okay. This often unspoken paradox is one of the reasons why few consultants are effective, and why many clients openly criticize, sue, or resent their consultant.

A consultant is anyone from whom information or influence is requested. When you read this book, you're asking to be influenced. When you ask for directions from the gas station attendant he becomes a consultant. When you ask your wait person whether the soup of the day is good, you've turned an order taker into a consultant. Similarly, when patients come to you asking for help with a health complaint and you use your influence and communication skills to shape the outcome, you are a consultant too. Any consultant will tell you one of the greatest challenges is to get the client to accept the advice and make a change.

When doctors hire a consultant to dislodge the status quo or help bail themselves out of a lack of new patients or poor compliance, they are asking to be influenced. Do people change? Slowly. Kicking. And complaining loudly about the new, and at first, uncomfortable procedure or perspective.

Just remember the advice you're getting is merely someone's opinion. No one can predict the future and every consultant makes mistakes. Witness the countless times you've gotten lost after someone says "you can't miss it," or the times you've wondered what anyone saw in cream of rutabaga soup!

There are several techniques you can use to size up a consultant's suggestions. Run through this list when you're confronting some advice that seems uncomfortable at first:

Blaming you: This is the easiest of consultant ploys. Lack of new patients? It's your fault. Can't get your patient visit average above 22 visits? That's your fault. You have high staff turnover? That's your fault too, doctor. In fact, every problem in your office is your fault because other doctors using the same technique, who went to the same school, and practice in the same town aren't having any problems. So it must be you.

What is so convenient about rendering this kind of advice is that it's almost always true. It *is* the doctor's fault. But confronting the doctor in this way rarely results in change. However, it is the safest observation that can come from the comfortable Herman Miller desk of a consultant who somehow feels equipped to diagnose your problem over the telephone. Without visiting your office he or she miss hearing the X-ray room dialogue, seeing you stumble through a report of findings, and hundreds of other details. A consultant must be willing to get his or her hands dirty! Before accepting any advice from any consultant it's important that they actually see the context of the problem. Otherwise expect cookie-cutter solutions and suggestions based on someone else's personality, value system, or vision of the future.

Specific action plan: Ever watch one of those movie review TV shows? You can tell these movie selection consultants love their work, jetting to Cannes and mingling with Hollywood's elite. They seem to wield a tremendous amount of influence with their weekly critique of directors, actors, and screen writers.

If you've ever bucked their reviews and seen one of their "thumbs down" picks and enjoyed it, you start questioning their other recommendations. Eventually you'll reach the same conclusion I have. These types of shows are really just entertainment and serve no other purpose except to publicize the latest movies playing on postage stamp-sized screens at the mall!

Oh, it's easy for consultants to sit on the sidelines and judge others, but what specific suggestions do they have for improvement? Can they offer a step-by-step action plan that accepts where the client is today and can get them to where they want to be? Simply casting blame without a constructive "here's what I'd do" plan for change is merely a judgment call of little value.

"I don't know:" A consultant's willingness to admit they don't have all the answers is an important dimension of their character. Even a 20-year veteran of the trenches can't have all the answers. A jack of all trades is usually the master of none. Be careful of any consultant who promises to organize your front desk, sell you adjusting tables, and motivate you and your staff at regular sessions in the hotel ballroom for a single monthly payment!

Providing holistic advice is probably the most effective type of consulting and that usually means being willing to refer. In the same way patients start doubting the recommendations of a doctor who proclaims to be an expert on back pain, nutrition, weight loss, body building, mattress selection, ergonomics, and water purification, be suspicious of one-stop supermarkets for your practice. Some foresighted consulting firms have financial planners and psychologists on staff, but most do not.

Walk the talk: You'd die laughing if you saw behind the scenes at many of the practice management consultant's offices. Like the false fronts of a Hollywood back lot, most consulting firms are as disorganized as the clients they profess to be able to help!

In offices of the rare exceptions you'll see focus, planning, and attention to detail. Before signing up or accepting the advice of any consultant, visit their offices. Show up unannounced and check out the desk tops, bulletin boards, and the general tone of the office. Ask yourself if what you see is what you want for your office. How do they handle scheduling, last minute changes, or your surprise visit? Are they an example of the type of organization, staff relationships, and internal communication systems you want?

When patients show up in your office they are checking the congruency of your consulting advice too. And while they might not put on white gloves to test for dust on the chrome parts of your adjusting table, they are sizing up countless details about your office, your appearance, your staff, your communications, your personality, and your recommendations. They'll never tell you that they'd be more compliant if you'd lose 20 pounds or that they'd refer their friends if you didn't practice in a pig pen. That's what their subconscious tells them. When a patient comes into your office and asks to be influenced, you become a consultant, facing many of the same challenges the consultants you've hired face.

Patients cling to a medical model of health for the same reason doctors cling to outdated procedures. Patients fail to comply with home care for the same reasons doctors fail to follow their own personal fitness program. And patients decide not to refer their friends to your office for many of the same reasons you don't refer your friends to join your practice management firm.

When you start thinking like the consultant you are, you discover there's more to chiropractic than simply improving a patient's spinal biomechanics. That's the relatively easy part. The challenge is in presenting change in such a way that it will be more attractive and safer than the status quo. The success and personal fulfillment promised in a career of service to others comes by not blaming others, but by providing a specific action plan, and having the willingness to admit you don't have all the answers, and walking the talk.

How does it feel to be a consultant? ■

BUILDING VERSUS GROWING

The ads in the professional newspapers simultaneously excite and depress me. At one end of the spectrum you'll find the wild abandon resembling the untamed western frontier. At the other end is the crass double-your-income ads that suggest that making money is the highest calling in chiropractic. And while I don't advocate a life of ashes and sack cloth, seeing the ads pandering to the lowest common denominator alarms me. What if patients saw these publications!

Of special interest to me has been the ads from practice management firms that offer practice building techniques at their seminars and pricey telephone consulting sessions. I've always been intrigued as to how these organizations could continue to exist, and what prompted practitioners to sign up for these expensive, dependency-creating arrangements. Lack of self-esteem? Isolation? Low confidence? As I've met more and more doctors who have admitted to, and enjoyed their practice management relationship, my attitudes have become more tolerant.

What I've learned is that most practice management firms have an honest interest in helping doctors attain the success and fulfillment they deserve. Yet, as a non-D.C., the ploys used to get doctors to "reenlist" and make doctors seemingly dependent upon the consultant seem self-serving. Instead of being a mentor and facilitator, all too many consultants become an expensive habit, fueled by self-doubt and an inferiority complex.

The key is to look for a consultant who is more interested in helping you "grow" your practice rather than someone interested in helping you "build" your practice. The distinction deserves some further explanation.

When contractors "build" a building they orchestrate a symphony of building materials, laborers, and time schedules to create something that wasn't there before. Contractors and subcontractors take dissimilar materials and create something new—usually the vision of an architect or planner. Lots of diesel fuel, electricity, talent and muscle power are needed to fashion these various raw materials into a usable structure. While the final result may not perfectly reflect the intended vision of the architect, it's important to note that whatever building emerges when the final cleaning crew leaves, it is the result of a new combination of materials that do not normally arrange themselves in this new way by the forces of nature. Not that we should scorn any structure other than caves and other natural shelter formations, but that the act of "building" invites, or most often requires, the flaws of an educated intelligence to design and assemble the parts. The result may be elegant or pedestrian.

Growth, on the other hand, as in growing a practice, is much more likely to offer more satisfying qualities. While buildings don't "grow," a practice can. One of the fundamentals of anything that can grow, is that it is alive and in good health (100% function).

A practice does not grow when the doctor is not healthy. A practice does not grow if the staff is not healthy. A practice does not grow when the office is not healthy (procedures, relationships, communications, etc.). Plants, animals, and practices flourish when they are healthy.

Do you have a healthy practice? If it's not growing, better check its vital signs. According to *Dorland's Medical Dictionary*, health is defined as "optimum physical, mental, and social well-being and not merely the absence of disease or infirmity." What does that mean when applied to a chiropractic office?

Physical

What does your office look like to an anxious, apprehensive new patient? Is it organized? Does it function properly? Can it adapt to a changing environment, or is it stuck with policies and procedures that served you five years ago? Is it efficient? Are patients walking down hallways in examination gowns? Is the doctor putting in 15 miles walking between a half dozen adjusting rooms and wasting valuable time? Do patients have to climb steps? Do patients have to apologize to friends about the outdated office colors? Is the office in a good location? Can patients find adequate parking? Form follows function and without the proper form, your office cannot function (health) properly.

Mental

This is the key. Like health, that is an inside job, your mental condition controls your practice. Your practice will never outgrow your self-esteem or clinical self-confidence. When you explore the upper reaches of professional sports, even the most physical (weight lifting for example), you discover it is primarily a mental game. Ever watch the expressions on the faces of Olympic athletes moments before their competition? It's a brain game. Those who can harness their brains best are most likely to win.

Still blaming insurance companies, patients, weather, geography, or your college chemistry instructor? You're wasting time. It's in your head. If there are cluttered closets in your brain, there are cluttered closets in your practice. If you don't have high standards and an attention to detail in your own thinking, then you probably don't expect much of your staff or patients. It's you. You are your practice. And it all starts inside the most powerful organ of your body. Is the practice healthy? Just examine the mental condition of the doctor. The rest follows.

Social

In a chiropractic setting, social well-being addresses the relationships between staff, doctor, and patients. When working with chiropractic assistants in an in-office consulting situation, it is quite revealing how they refer to their relationship with the doctor. Staff members who work "with" Dr. SoAndSo find the relationship more satisfying than staff members who work "for" the doctor.

The other critical social relationship that affects the health of the practice is the doctor/patient relationship. Here, the doctor's communication skills shape the health of the social (and clinical) relationship with patients. Doctors who neglect to over-communicate suffer from poor compliance and a lack of referrals.

Besides explaining the nature and severity of their problem, one of the primary purposes of over-communication is to make sure patients know it's their problem, not yours. Because of your training and first hand clinical experience it's easy to forget that patients don't automatically appreciate the significance of their aberrant spinal biomechanics. Or more frustrating, that patients don't value their health as much as you do. Relentless communications and singleness of purpose are essential for defining the social contract you have with your patients. Only when patients "own" their problem and appreciate its significance are they likely to make better decisions about their care in your office.

Fees, personality, grooming habits, scheduling, waiting time, and bedside manner are other factors that shape the social dimension of a healthy practice. Overlooking any of these complex social dynamics can result in a variety of practice pathologies. Bringing in an outsider to "build" your practice is not likely to help until interferences to the natural growth process are removed. If your practice has plateaued (not merely the absence of disease or infirmity), the natural growth process has been shunted. A vital, healthy practice grows until some barrier or limiting force is encountered. It is the role of an ethical consultant to help diagnose this limiting force and set free the natural growth process.

While *growing* your practice may take longer then *building* your practice, the results are more lasting. What if the dreamy promises practice "builders" came true? What would you do if twenty new patients were milling around your front door next Monday morning when you drove up? Chances are your current procedures would make more than half of them angry because of waiting too long. The rushed (or nonexistent) report of findings would sabotage the relationship for still others who wouldn't understand the what, how, and why of chiropractic.

Building a bigger practice could be toxic. Growing a practice allows for assimilation, evolution, and adaptation. Building is short term. Growing is long term. Building is mechanistic. Growing is vitalistic—like chiropractic. ■

IF I RAN
THE ZOO

Like sharks, which biologists believe have not changed much in the millions of years of their existence, many of the practice management firms that cruise the waters of the profession, have remained unchanged too. All too many are still beating the dead horse of insurance, focusing much of their "management" advice on increasingly clever schemes to extract ever dwindling amounts of money available from insurance companies.

Like many, I believe this impending "insurance crisis" will ultimately be a positive thing for chiropractic. It will tend to weed out some of those who got involved in the profession for the wrong reasons. It will serve to dissuade those from practicing who do not have a strong understanding, trust, and philosophical basis in chiropractic. Watch for lots of used equipment (and practices) for sale in the near future. This is a time to watch your overhead and be smart about not incurring new debt.

The real tragedy will be the students. Rip Van Winkle never had it this bad! After a few short years of schooling, students are entering a much different practice environment than when they began school. What impact will large loan balances have on the fledgling new practitioners?

If I ran a practice management firm and was sensitive to the pressures and cultural trends chiropractic is facing today, I'd do things a little differently. For current practice management firms that need some fresh ideas, or a new upstart company that wants to command a presence, here are some free ideas:

Creating a nondependency relationship: Like the highest calling of any doctor (to prevent what he or she treats), tomorrow's practice management firms must work hard at keeping the relationship short. If a doctor simply wants to belong to a group, that can be accommodated through some type of mastermind or "alumni" group with a per-attendance fee. The objective should be to help doctors "get it" and not see how many years they can be strung along.

Telling the truth: It seems so basic. Like chiropractic that corrects the cause, chiropractic management should look to correct cause. Almost always the cause is the doctor. Tomorrow's practice management firm will have psychological experts and counseling services to help facilitate breakthrough changes in the doctor. At the root of virtually every practice management problem is the doctor.

Clearly stated value system: The chameleon-like appearance of most practice management firms makes it difficult to know just what value system will be taught. Like doctors who are afraid to reveal too much of their own identity for fear they may offend someone, today's management firms submerge key values in the hopes of being more attractive to more people. Oh sure, if you dig deep enough you can find the Jewish management firm, the Christian management firm, the nice guy management firm, the just-love-and-serve-them-enough management firm, the positive mental attitude management firm, etc. That's not good enough. Tomorrow's management firm will need a clearly stated mission statement, philosophy statement, and spiritual statement of beliefs so doctors will know exactly what they're buying. And there will be no pulling punches! If you're spiritual life is a mess, your life and your practice is a mess.

Set measurable outcomes: Incredibly, this is a missing element in many management relationships. Often, merely a small rise in statistical amounts of new patients, volume, or profit serves as a goal. Too bad. Like many patients who feel worse before they get better, or need care without obvious symptoms, quantitative statistics aren't sufficient. How do you want it to be after a six month or one year stint with your management company? How long are you willing to withhold judgment before crying foul? How are you going to measure your psychological satisfaction level? What will constitute a "successful" relationship? What are you really buying? The bottom line is accountability. Without some form of mutually agreed-upon outcome, the relationship can lose focus and result in misunderstanding.

Trusted coach: If all we had to do was read a book or hear a "solution" at a seminar and instantly adopt it, personal and practice development would be a snap. And very inexpensive. The days of "just do this" are gone. What most of us really need is a coach that will provide physical, mental, and spiritual support as we try out new success habits. This is crucial because many success habits feel uncomfortable at first. It takes a good coach (not just someone who was successful years ago) to inspire, motivate, challenge, cajole, and beg us to adopt an idea or procedure which makes us at first feel insecure and awkward. A coach must allow rejection and failure, yet nurture an environment in which new ideas can be tested in safety. This requires small group settings and the help of talented facilitators—not sitting in a hotel ballroom with hundreds of other participants!

Chiropractic philosophy: Let's not forget why we're here! Without a constant dose of chiropractic philosophy, it's too easy to lose sight of the real purpose for being in practice, and forget what unites all chiropractic doctors. This philosophy not only should be talked about, but also practiced. Virtually everything from the registration process to the post-seminar mailings should be true to the chiropractic philosophy. No symptom treating! Seminars should start on time. No excuses about outside forces such as geographical location or economic times should be tolerated. No finger pointing.

Tribal connections: Small group mentoring should be encouraged. Simply having a toll-free number to call a consultant isn't enough. Each doctor should have a number of peers out in the trenches whom they can call on a more regular and low-key basis. These small tribal units could be used to help avoid the sense of isolation many doctors feel. Additionally, they provide a ready source of problem-solving brain power. This decentralized approach may sound threatening to the type of control normally exercised by traditional practice management firms today, but this is what it will take to provide the safety net needed for personal and practice growth.

Embrace diversity: Chiropractic is a profession of Lone Rangers; iconoclasts who embraced a profession they were told no one wanted or needed. This diversity should be honored. In the same way immigrants from around the world have improved the United States through cultural diversity, so too is chiropractic enriched. Without this diversity there is danger of in-breeding and losing touch with the world outside the chiropractic subculture. Participant feedback should be invited. No charismatic management group leader has all the answers. There is a wealth of wisdom in the audience. Coaching is a dialogue, not a monologue. Differences of opinion should be nurtured in the Socratic technique of uncovering the truth. Put microphones in the audience.

If you've found a practice management firm that has already implemented these suggestions, congratulations. If this mythical management firm I've described is impossible to create, so be it. The real purpose of these observations is to question the status quo. As times change, so too should the management advice rendered this profession. The good old boy, "this-is-the-way-we've-always-done-it" must change. The psychographic of the typical patient has changed, and so too must the rules of practice conduct.

Intelligence is defined as the ability to adapt. Certainly our ability to exist for long periods under the ocean, in the Arctic, or in space are shining examples of our intelligence. To make course corrections on our commute home by hearing traffic reports on the radio is the result of our intelligence. And changing one's expectations from practice management consultants as the world changes is a sign of intelligence, too. ■

DANGEROUS
OPPORTUNITY

Fueled by blind ambition, a desire to change the world, or misled by thinking success could be measured statistically, doctors in the 1980s squandered a valuable opportunity to dramatically change the perception and utilization of chiropractic. Prevalent insurance, combined with low deductibles, made chiropractic accessible to millions of people who might not have otherwise considered it. Instead of using this great influx as an opportunity to inspire and educate patients, it became expensive houses, polyester leisure suits, Rolex watches, and leveraged lifestyles.

Why waste valuable clinical time educating patients that chiropractic is bigger than mere pain relief? Why invest energy in patient education when there were countless other $100 deductibles just waiting in the wings if they could be enticed into the office?

Too many doctors ate their "seed corn" of the future.

Those days are gone. Today at seminars, state conventions, and other gatherings of chiropractors where there is talk of the future, it's done in hushed tones, punctuated by loud "everything's-okay-at-our-house" affirmations.

"How's it going Dr. Bob?" he asks slapping an old friend on the back with a forced grin.

"A little down, John. You?" goes the reply, mustering his most confident posture.

You can almost hear the shallow breathing and feel the sweaty palms over the phone. "Bill, what's going on out there? You've got your ear to the ground, what's the future looking like?"

Where do you start? Do you remind them of the calls I get from doctors congratulating themselves on their best year ever? Or should I join them for a few tears in their beer? There is change in the air. And it's making many doctors nervous. You can smell it.

The word "change" in Japanese comes from joining two ideograms together, much like a contraction or compound word. Combine the ideograms meaning "dangerous" and "opportunity" and you have the Japanese word for change. Change can be dangerous, but it can also be an exciting opportunity. Since the only tangible thing remaining from the change afforded by easy access to chiropractic care in the 1980s is countless files with brightly colored labels on them, how are you preparing for the inevitable and next dangerous opportunity, the disappearance of insurance cases.

While no one can predict the future, here are a couple of different scenarios postulated by doctors and influencers I've encountered in the profession:

The Denial Scenario: If Alfred E. Newman was a chiropractor, this would be his outlook. The "What Me Worry?" approach combines a sense of naiveté with the classic frog in the beaker metaphor. Remember? Put a frog in a beaker of water and slowly heat the water and the frog will adapt to the increasingly warmer water until it boils to death. But drop the frog into the warm water and he quickly jumps out.

In chiropractic the warm water started out by first taking insurance assignment, hiring staff to handle the insurance "department", then computers, increasingly more complex software to shake the checks loose, seminars, fax machines, electronic filing; by now the water's beyond tepid. Worse, care recommendations are increasingly dictated by state legislatures that cap visit amounts, or unsuccessful chiropractors selling out to insurance companies, by passing judgment on the care rendered by their chiropractic brethren!

When a profession starts "eating" its own, you know there's something terribly wrong.

Those who deny there is a problem, figure that someone else will solve it, remain on the course they've set for themselves, and wait for the crowd to indicate which path to take.

The Hard Worker Scenario: This is a less naive version of the Denial outlook. Here, the doctor recognizes there is a problem, probably a serious one, but the strategy for dealing with it isn't ignorance, it's simply working harder.

Sadly, many practice management organizations are still beating this dying horse, continuing to counsel their clients to simply do more of what used to work. With every delaying strategy and claim-cutting tactic the insurance companies employ, they respond with thicker narratives, new CPT codes, and other gamesmanship. Alternative sources of income are seriously explored, as areas of the office start looking like a health food store or a gymnasium!

Whether they recognize it or not, the conclusion the Hard Worker reaches is that you can't make a living in chiropractic. Self doubt, burn out, and a self-fulfilling prophesy lurk around the corner. Suddenly, they discover it isn't the A.M.A. that will destroy chiropractic, it's the insurance industry.

The Waiting For Santa Claus Scenario: This is a popular outlook among doctors who have never actually talked with their Canadian peers to the north, and think some form of nationalized health care will solve all their problems. Administered by the federal government and funded by some phantom source of tax dollars, proponents of this approach reveal their blind trust in the same folks who hatched Medicare!

In light of the recent abuse it has received at the hands of legislatures in an increasing number of states, it's hard to know for sure how chiropractic will fare. But it's not likely to be the dreamy vision of sugar plum fairies that dance in the minds of children waiting for Santa's arrival.

Regardless of what happens, just remember they'll call it health care, but what they will really be talking about is sickness care. Even in a best case scenario, chiropractic will probably be limited to 12 visits for the "natural" relief of low back pain much like that sanctioned by the RAND study. Then the next logical step after that is to get it eliminated all together or teach "real" doctors to do it at weekend seminars!

The Opportunity Scenario: Many doctors will find this new practice environment a source of excitement and recommitment. It will require self-confidence and a willingness to make mistakes. There are no history books to consult when predicting what will happen as the insurance industry reorganizes and we see more and more patients without insurance and $1000 or higher deductibles the rule rather than the exception.

If all insurance disappeared tomorrow, what would be the cost of an adjustment? Certainly not in the 90th percentile as currently surveyed by *Fee Facts*! How would that affect your income? Your lifestyle? Your overhead? Your focus?

Get accustomed to something called "downward mobility." Instead of striving for more, we will find a new sense of purpose and fulfillment from simplicity. The debt-laden lifestyles of the past will remain in the past. People are paying off their credit cards and avoiding incurring more debt—even with low Roosevelt-era interest rates. Patients will likely wait longer and be worse off when initially consulting your office. It will require better patient education than ever before.

There will be plenty of offices that will survive and thrive in this new world. Just as there were hugely successful practices before insurance, there will be hugely successful practices when it is gone. Will yours be one of them?

Which scenario or combination do you think will happen? Better yet, what are you doing today to lay the groundwork for successfully bridging this dangerous opportunity? Because change happens. For some it means going kicking and screaming, holding onto the past. For others, with a strong chiropractic philosophy, excellent patient education efforts, low overhead, and a technique that allows them to easily and effectively serve their patients, the future is already in place. What's your plan? ■

THE DECENTRALIZATION
OF CHIROPRACTIC

John Naisbitt (*Megatrends*) referred to it as decentralization. Faith Popcorn (*The Popcorn Report*) called it cocooning. Whatever the nomenclature, what these two accurate soothsayers of the future agree on, is that as a culture we tend to be moving away from institutions and central authority and towards separatism, diversity, and a sense of turning inward. The "me" generation of the 80s has become the "free" generation of the 90s. More and more people are less willing to define themselves by what group they belong to, the things they buy, or the beliefs they hold.

The trendsetters of our culture who have the resources to act on these feelings, first moved to seaside Malibu to escape the oppression of L.A. When that lost its uniqueness, the Rocky Mountains of Aspen became the magnet. Now Montana and Idaho seem isolated enough to reflect this urge to drop out of the mainstream. Who knows the next locale that will appeal to the desire to escape.

The trend called cocooning, which plays heavily into Popcorn's observations can be seen in the recent rise in videotape rentals and decline in movie theater attendance. More and more restaurants are offering delivery and take out service. Microwave popcorn and home security systems are growth industries. More and more people are finding it unsafe or unsavory to go out. Instead they're staying home. Products and services that are growing are often those that reflect this growing sensitivity to matters of family, security, and local convenience. Home remodeling is in. Buying a bigger house is out. Pizza delivery is in. Eating out is out. Savings accounts are in. Foreign aid is out.

At a time when the United Sates is thought of as the only super power and the policeman of the world, we want to turn inward and protect our jobs and educate our children at home. An isolated superpower is an oxymoron. What's it going to be?

These same attitudes are being felt in the area of health care. The centralization of health care (hospitals) are losing out (or spawning) the highly popular "doc in a box." Hospital administrations, seeing the trend, are now getting into the business themselves, claiming the best of both worlds; "neighborhood convenience backed up by the largest hospital in the city..." The message is clear: adapt or die. A growth sector for today's hospitals? Same-day outpatient surgeries.

Perhaps pharmaceuticals are the most decentralized of all. Yes, they are initially purchased at a centralized location, but as a treatment, most drugs and medicines are highly portable. They can be taken into the cocoon. If you're unable, many pharmacies have a delivery service. Perfect!

How does chiropractic fare in this new cultural order? Does chiropractic need to make changes to adequately respond or take advantage of this new reality? You decide.

Like elective, same-day surgeries, patients must go to a somewhat centralized location. Your office. Fortunately for you, your office is probably more convenient, located in a safe suburb instead of a decaying downtown location. However, unlike drugs, chiropractic cannot be stored up or easily transported. In chiropractic there is simultaneous production and consumption. It can never be a commodity—it is a service. Domino's can store up pizzas, but Domino's can't store up its delivery!

Because this is an uncharted area, some of these ideas may sound impractical, expensive, or inappropriate. That's all right because after all, who can really predict the future?

Location: Location is taking on a new meaning. The question isn't just drive-by traffic count and zoning laws affecting clinic signage, but are you in a growing or a decaying neighborhood. Prospective patients are judging you based on the character of your office location. Sadly, the inner city is often being left to the disenfranchised and those who cannot afford to move out.

Accessibility: The Southland Corporation, owner of the chain of 7-11 convenience stores, describes optimum accessibility as "on the right, right on the way home." They are the masters of accessibility. This is a further refinement of the location aspect. Not only must your office be located in the right neighborhood, it has to be easy to get to. Parking is more of a factor affecting compliance than many doctors recognize. Many patients size up the number of cars in your parking lot and drive right on by. They know that lots of cars means a long wait. Instant gratification is in. Waiting is out.

Hours: Related to accessibility, your hours of operation reveal a lot about you. Countless dentists have built successful practices serving patients between 6:00 A.M. and 9:00 A.M. or 5:00 PM to 11:00 P.M. If you're in a suburb or bedroom community to a large city, consider trying some extreme hours. Are you an early riser? How about 5:30 A.M. to 10:00 A.M. once or twice a week?

Lighting: Parking lot safety is an issue critical to all offices during the winter months. Then, even the most mainstream office hour arrangement can mean that patients are leaving your office in the dark. Ask your staff and a handful of trusted female patients if they perceive your office as safely lit.

Noon lay lectures: Not wanting to leave the cocoon at night or to be delayed in getting there, consider lunch time spinal care classes. Encourage patients to bring a friend from the office. Serve a light lunch or fruit tray. Come up with alternatives to the 6:30 P.M. health talk.

House calls: More and more medical doctors are reviving this "new" idea from a previous generation. In the same way few patients will trouble you at home if you offer your number, few will take advantage of this extraordinary gesture. Offer anyway. It makes an important statement about your accessibility and sense of caring. (Of course it costs the patient more. But cost isn't always the issue—quality and convenience is.)

New Patient Information: Help make it easy for people still at home to get to know you and decide if you are what they need or want.

Help them "pre-qualify" themselves. Put together an information packet about your office. Introduce yourself and reveal your motives for getting involved in chiropractic. Share your health attitude and your mission. Explain what generally happens on the first couple of visits. Include some simple home screening tests that would suggest the value of an in office visit. The goal is to put a prospective patient at ease and help lure them out of the security of their cocoon. Of course, let your current patients know you have this information so they can tell others about it!

Home care: While an adjustment isn't easily transportable like a bottle of pills, exercises and certain other adjunctive procedures are. This doesn't mean 100% of your patients will comply, however it helps patients feel they are in control and participating in their own recovery. Give every patient something they can do at home, even if it is as simple as sleeping with the right type of pillow or doing some simple exercises.

Some of these ideas are old ones. Others may push you beyond your comfort zone or don't seem to make sense where you practice. Just remember the world is changing. Simply doing more of what used to work is no guarantee of success in the future. Read John Naisbitt's books. Read *The Popcorn Report*. Read Alvin Toffler's *Future Shock*. Read Ken Dychtwald's *Age Wave*. Find out what people who are on the lookout for business and industry are thinking about the future. And then ultimately recognize that the easiest way to predict your own future is to invent it. ■

LOW TECH HEALTH IN A HIGH TECH WORLD

Is chiropractic too low tech for today's scientific-high-tech oriented individual? Perhaps. Not only from our early childhood when we are introduced to the medical model of health, but everyday, we often look outside our bodies for the keys to health and happiness. It starts in the morning when we crave the first cup of coffee and sugary Danish to get us going, and continues until evening with a drink to "relax us." When you take up the anti-medicine cause, realize you're also taking on the anti-coffee, anti-sugar, anti-alcohol, and anti-anything that is used as a "drug."

Yet crusading "against" anything is usually a waste of time. More success is usually found crusading "for" something. Campaigning for sexual equality is likely to have more impact than fighting against sexual harassment. Helping people to read will have more effect than a drive to obliterate illiteracy. One is directional and resourceful, the other is whiny and judgmental. If chiropractic is to assume its rightful place and become more accepted by the baby boom population, we must concentrate on being *for* chiropractic and not merely against medicine. Yet without much of the technology that has made palliative approaches seem "real" and "scientific," chiropractic must consider new ways to communicate its unique and unduplicated approach to today's health-conscious generation.

If you've ventured into any of B.J. Palmer's green books, you'll get a glimpse of a mid-twentieth century awe of the body. To recognize that we each have the inborn potential to be healthy (proper function) if there isn't any interference (subluxation), is a low-tech idea that had considerable more appeal before the wonder drugs and exotic surgical interventions we see today. To discover that each of us has "it" and that all we need to do is unlock "it" through normalizing spinal biomechanics may be too simplistic for many today. Where are the gadgets? Where are the dials? Where are the effortless injections? Where is the "better world through chemistry" that we've been taught?

Making low-tech chiropractic attractive to a generation that sent a man safely to the moon and back again is the real challenge facing the advancement of the profession. Some say "fight fire with fire" and have crusaded for more chiropractic research. Certainly this is a worthy cause, yet the fundamental question isn't, "Does chiropractic work?" Chiropractic has been working since the beginning. And results are not enough either. With its enviable success record over the last 100 years, there should be lines in front of every chiropractic office. Clearly, incredible, non-invasive, affordable, conservative results are not enough.

Obviously the necessary mind-shift has to start with the doctor and his or her own lifestyle and be exhibited by the staff before patients will take chiropractic as seriously as we do. Yet, you'd be surprised how many doctors have their own children vaccinated ("Just to be sure"). Or drink coffee ("It's my only vice"). Or only get adjusted a couple times a year ("I'm too busy"). Or worse, still smoke ("I just can't seem to quit").

When the doctor sells out, even a little, it's reflected in the type of staff he or she surrounds themselves with. How many countless offices employ staff members who, even after a couple years on the job, still haven't been adjusted? Sure, the rationalizations come easy. "It's too hard to find someone around here" or "I don't want to confront my staff" or "It's just a job and they won't be around long anyway."

By the time this "we're-not-really-that-serious-about-chiropractic" message is received by patients, chiropractic is positioned as merely a natural form of aspirin one considers as a last resort before surgery.

Breaking through this ingrained mind-set that a typical new patient brings to your office is pivotal in growing patients that ultimately adopt a chiropractic lifestyle. Here are some conversation starters that might help patients get in touch with the marvelous bodies they are residing in and see chiropractic in a powerful new way:

The ultimate drug factory: Share with your patients the incredible system their bodies have to manufacture adrenalin, digestive enzymes, and hormones in the correct strength and quantity and deliver them quickly and perfectly where they are needed. Give your patients the awareness to ask themselves why someone would need antacids for their stomach or cough medicine in response to the commercials they see on TV.

Getting replacement parts: This is a great topic to discuss if the subject of cancer comes up in conversation in the adjusting room. Explain to patients how quickly different parts of their bodies are being replaced with new cells. We each have a new stomach lining in a matter of hours. New liver tissue in a matter of months. New bones in a matter of years. Ask them what they think controls this cell replication process. Ask them what might cause these cells to create a mutant replacement.

Is it dead or alive? What's the difference between tissue that is alive and tissue that is dead? Most patients have never thought about this one. We take for granted that we're alive, but have rarely thought about what separates us from those who have just departed. Help patients honor their bodies and appreciate the role of the nervous system in its maintenance.

How to catch a cold: Most patients would rather not have a "common cold" yet have never thought about why they don't automatically get one when exposed to someone who does. Ask your patients what they could do to purposely catch a cold or any other disease. Show the connection to the nervous system.

The parable of the deadly dinner: My favorite is Dr. Riekeman's story of a man who has eaten a poorly prepared meal and finds himself throwing up several hours later. Ask your patients (or staff!) if the person throwing up is sick or well. Then ask them the possible consequences of taking a drug to prevent throwing up! Emphasize the role of proper function (controlled by the nervous system) in the regaining and maintenance of good health.

Would you rather feel good or be healthy? This is a wonderful conversation starter for certain patients. Most people weaned on a medical model of health would prefer to feel good. Or, at least get through life with as little pain as possible. Remind patients of what the first symptom of heart disease or hypertension usually is. Your discussion naturally returns to the role of the nervous system in maintaining proper function. Help your patients understand why chiropractic doctors are so interested in the spine (the movable covering of the nervous system most often the source of interference).

Your first cells: Ask your patients what they think the first differentiated cells in their bodies were when they were growing in the womb. Many patients will think it was the heart because of the tremendous emphasis our culture has placed on this circulatory muscle. Show pictures of early embryonic development in the photography of Lennart Nilsson. Help patients see the importance of organization and nervous system control.

It's unlikely you'll get enough patients to attend chiropractic college like you did so they can fully appreciate chiropractic. The best offices (run by the best communicators) recognize their role as teachers and give their patients the equivalent of *Cliff Notes* so they can better understand what you do—so they'll do what you do.

Sadly, even your best patients probably still "believe" in medicine. Help them discover there is no Santa Claus. Explain that doctors can't heal the body. Show them why outside solutions that merely treat the symptoms don't work and are probably counterproductive. Better yet, let them know *they* are Santa Claus! ■

HOW DO
YOU FEEL?

I encounter chiropractors completely inside the medical model of health care (sickness care) who look at me suspiciously when I reveal that I try to get adjusted about once a week. These are the same doctors who are proud of the fact that they can work pain relief miracles with their patients in as few as six or ten visits. These are the chiropractors who look down with disdain on their brethren who "keep patients coming back" even after their insurance has been exhausted. These are chiropractors who can't understand offices crowded with children and non-symptomatic adults. Chiropractors who think symptomatic relief is the sole purpose of chiropractic. Chiropractors who may not fully appreciate the confining view of chiropractic they have created for themselves.

Doctors who think otherwise, and yearn for their patients to adopt a chiropractic lifestyle, are often frustrated that patients depend upon how they feel to judge whether they need to continue seeking chiropractic care.

During the heady days of $100 deductibles, this was less of a concern for many doctors. Then, the objective was to get as many new patients as possible and enjoy the escalating fees insurance companies would pay for adjustments, modalities, and X-rays. This is when advertising, spinal exams, mall shows, and countless other promotional gimmicks were employed to entice as many insurance cases as possible into the office.

Bragging at chiropractic gatherings centered around new patient statistics.

This "sucking up" to the insurance industry, with its symptom-oriented measurement of health, set the stage for the current erosion chiropractic is experiencing at the hands of HMO and PPO proliferation. Not only did the coverage of sickness care insurance policies suggest that "feeling better" was a reason to discontinue care, but so did a lifetime of living in our treat-the-symptom" culture. Even with the millions of patients helped with low back pain and headaches in the last 10 years, how many would picket the county jail in protest if, like the 1930s, you were incarcerated for "practicing medicine without a license?"

Yet, when you suggest to patients that they can't trust how they feel, you enter dangerous territory. What is more fundamental than believing what we each feel?

It starts when we are children. We are taught that certain parts of our bodies are unclean. We are rewarded with sweets for good behavior. We develop a taste for certain kinds of food. We enjoy the feeling of riding a roller coaster or we avoid them—depending upon how we feel. Countless daily activities are performed based solely on how we feel.

"What do you feel like having for dinner tonight?"

Trusting how we feel has been ingrained into our behavior. For many, it is the only thing we *can* trust. It feels good to eat. Most of us stop eating when we are full and no longer feel like eating.

As our world becomes increasingly complicated and the harsh realities of being surrounded by, and depending upon technology we don't understand, feeling may be the last bastion of privacy. For most of us, everything from electronic garage door openers and CD players, to antibiotics and organ transplants take on an air of magic. We may not necessarily understand how they work, but we have an opinion about them!

Never mind the media is actively brainwashing us to feel certain ways about certain products, services, philosophies, and social concerns. Never mind there's no such thing as an unbiased reporter. Never mind that all too many of those in our culture are merely gratification orifices that consume, enjoy, discard, and search for more pleasure. The over-riding concern of all too many is to simply get through life by avoiding as much pain as possible. How you feel may not be as important as how you look, but it is certainly towards the top of most people's list.

Is it futile to try and explain to patients that they can't trust how they feel? You're asking them to go against one of the most fundamental ways they define themselves. The most self-confident and open-minded patients seem more willing to withhold judgment. Doctors who can project large amounts of conviction and trust are more effective in overcoming this dilemma. Those most familiar with chiropractic philosophy recognize that reframing the patients' perceptions about how they "feel" is an important component of the patient education process.

When you ask patients to stop trusting how they feel, it smacks of the Theory X school of thought made popular in the 1970s. It was held by some that you can't trust people, for when offered a choice they'll make the wrong one. The solution of course is to prevent the choice, eliminating failure. This authoritarian approach assumes a position 180 degrees opposite the overriding attitudes of the patients showing up in chiropractic offices today. You can't "manage" patients into compliance. You can't scare patients into compliance. You must coach patients to make better decisions. You have to honor the patient's decision and create a supportive environment.

We've all heard of the insurance salesmen who "just has our best interests at heart." We're immediately suspicious. And should be. Reach for your wallet to make sure it's still there!

At first glance one might assume that chiropractors are asking their patients to mistrust their bodies. On the contrary. Patients simply need better information so they can more accurately detect and interpret what they learn from their bodies. Here are some common health complaints that might offer opportunities for reframing:

Cutting your finger: Dr. Bernie Segal uses this metaphor. He exclaims how cutting his finger is an opportunity to witness the awe of the healing process. No one likes the feel of a cut finger, but seeing a bandaid on someone's finger is a chance to help them rethink their ideas about health and healing. "I see the same inborn force that controls your heart rate, digestion, and thyroid activity is healing your finger there..."

Headaches: It is estimated that at this very moment 25% of the population has a headache! Your patients may not tell you this but even some of your best patients still use aspirin. And if they don't, they certainly encounter family and friends who do. Imagine equipping your patients to observe when a work associate asks for aspirin, "What's wrong Bob, does your body have an aspirin shortage—again? When are you going to get at the cause of your headaches?"

Stomach aches: This is a perfect opportunity to teach your patients to ask why. It sounds something like this. "So Bob, why does your stomach hurt?" "I don't know, must have been something I ate." "Why do you think it was something you ate?" "It started hurting after I ate it." "Why do you think it hurts?" "Just sensitive, I guess." "Did everyone who ate the same thing you did get an upset stomach?" "No, I guess not." "Why do you suppose your stomach got upset and know one else's did?" "I don't know." The idea is to keep asking "why" until the person gets stuck. When that happens, it usually means they haven't thought about it before. It becomes a great opportunity to explain the role of the nervous system in maintaining proper function, etc.

First adjustment soreness: One reason many doctors don't call patients after their first adjustment is the fear that the patient may be actually doing worse. The patient may blame the doctor, so the doctor avoids what could be an important opportunity to astound the patient with exceptional service. "That discomfort you're feeling is a lot like... have you ever felt sore the morning after shoveling snow or raking leaves for the first time of the season? What you're feeling now is the same sort of thing; muscles which aren't used to supporting your spine in the proper way are probably just a little tired..." Unless you put the "blame" on the patient were it belongs, without an explanation patients incorrectly assume that it's your fault.

Wouldn't it be great if everyone learned about their bodies in an elementary school classroom in which basic physiology was taught with a "cause" philosophy instead of an "effect" orientation? Until it is, you have a responsibility to help your patients more accurately interpret the world around them. It's a big job. Do you feel up to it? ■

INTELLIGENT OR
MERELY SMART?

When Christopher Columbus "discovered" the new world he changed the way Europeans thought of the world. Now, over 500 years later, the reality of our spherical globe is obvious and rarely given a second thought. Yet imagine the huge numbers of Columbus' peers unwilling to accept this new model, clinging to their flat plate view of the world.

Columbus didn't return to the queen and her court and deliver a 15-minute report of findings explaining his discovery and get immediate acceptance! There were many advisors and leaders to convince. There were so many ingrained agendas to be protected. There were jobs to be safeguarded. Chains of command were threatened. The judgment and trust of religious officials came under scrutiny. There was considerable built-in resistance within the social and political order of the day that opposed any change.

Yet, with time, things changed. The leaders adapted and integrated this new truth into their thinking. Those who refused to adapt became anachronisms who lost their ability to influence and lead. Those who embraced, or at least were willing to "try on" the idea, survived and became part of the new order. (It is said that maturity is the ability to hold two opposing ideas in your mind simultaneously.) It is this same ability to adapt which is needed as chiropractic confronts change on many fronts.

In chiropractic circles it is a well accepted notion that the world is organized by a universal intelligence. Most of us call this force God. It is through this intelligence and by this intelligence that our bodies perform the millions of necessary functions to create, pump, and regulate our blood, digest nutrients, remove waste, and appropriately respond to the world around us. These functions are organized by the nervous system and work perfectly if there isn't any interference. Look up the definition of the word intelligence and you'll see a reference to the notion that intelligence is the "ability to adapt." It is our intelligence that permits us to adapt to new places, adapt to new ideas, and adapt to new ways.

Don't confuse intelligence with being smart. A lot of smart people aren't intelligent! A lot of intelligent people aren't very smart. The absent-minded professor who forgets where he put his car keys is almost a cliché. The inner city teenager with "street smarts" (the ability to adapt to his environment) is very intelligent even though he may not be able to read. Intelligence is a skill necessary for survival. Simply being smart can obscure the bigger picture and get one caught up in the minutia of the moment. It can even lead to extinction!

The full expression of an intelligent life is only possible as a result of an interference-free environment. We can ignore intelligence. We can cover it up. We can misinterpret it. We can deny it. But it is always there; immutable and perfect. For this universal intelligence to provide adaptation by providing a source of truth, there must be no interference. One of the most frequent sources of interference is in the feedback loop confirming previous action. Intelligence isn't a one-way expression, it constantly monitors the environment to insure that the intended outcome has been achieved. The brain sends the nerve impulse to the tissue, the tissue responds, and the tissue sends a nerve impulse back to the brain. As long as there isn't any interference in either direction, the homeostatic balance (adaptation) that allows us to function as we were designed, is permitted. Interfere with any part of this loop, the sending or the receiving and dysfunction results. Every time.

While this is a universal model to describe the function of living tissue, limiting this truth to human physiology overlooks the innumerable situations in which adaptability is so important. Is your management approach merely smart or truly intelligent?

Patient education: It's smart to have a systematized patient education program in your office, but it requires intelligence to assure that your patients understand the material. It takes intelligence to adapt the material or know when to provide supplementary information. It takes intelligence to make sure that the information you're communicating is relevant. Ask your patients how they describe chiropractic to others. Then use your intelligence to correct a patient's misinformed notions.

Changing insurance climate: It was probably smart to accept insurance because it allowed an affordable way for many patients to become introduced to chiropractic. However it isn't very intelligent to ignore the writing on the wall that plentiful insurance cases with low deductibles are almost gone. It is not intelligent to continue as if nothing has changed. While the first reaction may be one of denial, it takes intelligence to adapt. What would you do if insurance was gone tomorrow? Put in place the policies and procedures today that anticipate this eventuality.

Statistics: It is smart to keep statistics because they represent certain quantitative information about what has happened in the past. However your statistics aren't your practice, in the same way a map isn't the territory. It takes intelligence to interpret the data and create a suitable response. Better yet, are you tracking any "qualitative" statistics that can predict the direction of your quantitative statistics? Assign a number on an arbitrary scale of between 1 and 10 to monitor your personal satisfaction, energy level, and overall vitality. Track these daily and average them month to month and you'll see they are really the only statistics you need!

Office environment: It may be smart to keep a low overhead because it allows you to see a greater return on your investment. Yet in the long run it sabotages your success. If you intend to be in practice for more than a couple of years it would be more intelligent to invest in your practice. It takes intelligence to know when to update the colors, the furnishings, and the procedures to reflect changing tastes in our culture.

Staff: It may seem smart to pay your staff as little as possible, but it wouldn't be intelligent. Ultimately leading to high turnover, low salaries are often signs of the doctor's lack of respect for the staff. High turnover is among a patient's most frequent complaint about staff members. It raises concerns about the doctor and behind-the-scenes conduct that sabotages a patient's complete trust. A more intelligent approach would be to put yourself in your staff's shoes and see how difficult it is to give a high level of service to others if you're worried about how you're going to make ends meet.

Clearly, it's not an either/or situation. What's really required is a balance between being smart and being intelligent. When you combine the intelligent ability of adapting with the factual, pragmatic skills of being smart and add a good memory, you have something called wisdom.

Wisdom is one of the most valuable traits you can posses. It disappears when the ego renders us impatient or when we lack experience. It tells us when to yield and when to stand firm. It helps us identify principle and purpose.

Chiropractic needs doctors that are smart and chiropractic needs doctors that are intelligent. Today we especially need chiropractic doctors with wisdom. As we embark on a decade that will likely see the emergence of some form of socialized medicine, the rise of HMOs, and the elimination of all but catastrophic forms of insurance, chiropractic must seek the wisdom of chiropractic veterans. The health care revolution of the 1990's will require new levels of adaptation. It will require doctors who have a keen grip on chiropractic philosophy. Moreover, it will require intelligence to change, to modify and adapt this universal truth so that the influencers, the advisors, and the court of world opinion will accept and modify their world views. It will become a time of renaissance and discovery. Perhaps it will be the time when the public will finally discover a truth as fundamental as that of Columbus. ■

THE FIVE INGREDIENTS OF A WELLNESS PRACTICE

Imagine a practice in which patients begin care because of an ache or pain, get well, and remain under regular maintenance care program for the rest of their lives. Imagine a practice in which patients enter with a symptomatic and short term outlook about their health, discover what chiropractic is all about, and continue with wellness care while referring their friends and families. Imagine an office in which the doctor doesn't have a voracious appetite for new patients. For some offices an imagination isn't required. In these offices the doctor has the confidence and vision to adopt a long term vision of the future. In these offices the doctor is having a lot of fun.

Consulting with countless offices, I've discovered there are five basic reasons why patients don't remain in the office to continue wellness care. Which one of these reasons (or combination) is standing in your way of having a practice full of non-symptomatic families and children?

1. Results. It's safe to say that if you do not produce results during the initial pain-relief stages of chiropractic care, you will not earn the right to offer your patients wellness care. You must first give patients what they want (symptomatic improvement) before you are granted the opportunity to give them what they need (preventive wellness care). Fortunately for most doctors, even new doctors, symptomatic improvement is almost a foregone conclusion. Normalizing spinal biomechanics is almost certain to help the patient. While you help them with their symptomatic picture, you must slowly foreshadow the impending choice of continuing with a maintenance care.

2. Personality. If you have difficulty establishing patient rapport, it is unlikely to expect your partnership with a new patient to blossom into a long-term relationship. During the initial stages of care patients may put up with a doctor who seems distant or is less than enthusiastic so they won't have to start the process over somewhere else. Once patients are out of pain they leave the office. This is an especially hard aspect to diagnose. How do you tell a doctor that his or her lack of personality is the problem? Until personality transplants are perfected, appropriate tableside manners will continue to be a stumbling block for many doctors. Communicate your excitement about the body's ability to heal itself. Explain that the underlying muscles and soft tissues take longer to heal than indicated by the presence of symptoms. Review a couple of cases of patients who ride the roller coaster of getting well, dropping out when they feel better, only to have their problem soon return. Make this inevitable process understandable.

3. Patient Education. If you want patients to adopt a chiropractic lifestyle, you must give them a way to judge the necessity for their care beyond how they feel. A systematic, relentless patient education effort is necessary because of the pre-existing condition (medical model of health) that most patients have when they enter the office. Patient education is the only way to give patients a sufficient understanding of the nature and severity of their problem so they'll make better choices about their health. Besides motivating your patients, effective patient education pays off by giving them better ways of describing chiropractic, reasons for referring, and help for their defense of their chiropractic decision when they encounter skeptics. Without patient education even compliance for the sickness care portion of their case is difficult.

4. Time. Since chiropractic doctors rarely have to endure the 5:30 P.M. rush hour when they receive their maintenance care, this is somewhat difficult to appreciate. Patients are not living for a chance to be adjusted. They are getting adjusted so they can go out and live! If the waiting time in your office exacts too high a price on the lifestyles of your patients, you cannot expect them to continue coming in for care when they're feeling fine. And it's not just the waiting time in the reception room, it's the total elapsed time from when they get out of their car to the time they get back into their car (Door Slam Time). Have you ever measured how long patients are actually in your office during different times of the day?

5. Fees. Don't expect a practice full of maintenance care patients if wellness chiropractic care is too expensive. Even with the best patient education effort, it's unreasonable to think your patients will drive a less expensive car or forego a couple of dinners out with the kids, just so they can pay what you charge insurance companies for sickness care! This is another difficult aspect for most doctors to appreciate because they get their care for free, or at least without any impact to their monthly budget. Ask your best educated, once-a-month maintenance care patients you have now how often they'd come in if money were no object. Patients want what you have, but just can't afford it. Create a wellness fee policy for your office that makes continued preventive care affordable.

The lynch-pin in most offices is rarely just one of these points, but usually a combination of two or three. Until you hold a couple of patient focus groups and refine your communication feedback loop with your patients, efforts to establish a wellness practice will be a continuing source of frustration. ■

BEYOND THE
PINCHED NERVE

There was a time when chiropractic had to be presented simplistically because patients had little formal education, placed doctors on a pedestal, and were willing to comply simply because the doctor said to. Not so today. Today's baby boom generation is the most educated ever (25% have college degrees). They tend to question authority, and are increasingly seeking second opinions. The "pinched nerve" subluxation model of the past doesn't work like it used to.

Moreover, without a complete description and understanding of the nature and severity of their problem, patients don't take their condition seriously and ignore recommendations for the ongoing chiropractic lifestyle (maintenance care) necessary for the management of the chronic spinal problems many adults present.

The five components of the Vertebral Subluxation Complex accurately describe the multi-faceted condition that patients present in your office. It is a more accurate term than "subluxation" and "vertebral subluxation" presented to chiropractic patients and laughed at by medical doctors who have assailed the linguistics of the concept over the years.

The Vertebral Subluxation Complex as confirmed by medical researchers consists of spinal kinesiopathology (abnormal motion or position of spinal bones), neuropathophysiology (abnormal nervous system function), myopathology (abnormal muscle function), histopathology (abnormal soft tissue function), and pathophysiology (abnormal function of the spine and body). These five components occur simultaneously and are reduced with appropriate chiropractic care. There are six compelling reasons why this model should be presented to today's patients.

1. It's real. Review contemporary medical research and the physiological impact of aberrant spinal mechanics are revealed. While some of the researchers haven't used the identical terms used here, their description of these component parts correlate precisely.

Interestingly, in the recent attempts at merger between the ACA and the ICA, the respective parties *did* agree on the component basis of the Vertebral Subluxation Complex.

Sadly, chiropractic research is still suspect as a justification of chiropractic care. The medical community, which garners the most respect has already conducted the research affirming these five component parts. Review the books listed later for your own study and verification.

2. It overcomes the unscientific image of chiropractic. Chiropractic has been hurt by not having accepted scientific nomenclature to describe what chiropractic care does. The coronary patient can better describe a triple bypass heart surgery than most chiropractic patients can the purpose of their repeated visits!

The Vertebral Subluxation Complex takes patients beyond the notion of just a bone out of place. Using the names of the components as appropriate can linguistically substantiate the patient's perception that what's wrong with them has a name, is serious, and their Doctor of Chiropractic is knowledgeable in its treatment. Continuing to use the simplistic, vague, and non-scientific term of "subluxation" to refer to this multi-faceted condition undermines patient confidence. Today's patient, weaned on medical tests administered with the accuracy of three decimal places, yearns for a scientific basis to chiropractic.

Don't be put off thinking patients can't understand myopathology or histopathology! Ask any new patient what a hysterectomy, appendicectomy, or an electroencephalogram is and most can tell you, or at least they've heard of them before. These $50 words can help validate chiropractic to a group of patients who want assurance that they've made the right decision by consulting your office.

3. It provides a structure for your report of findings. The Vertebral Subluxation Complex supplies an organized structure for explaining to patients what's wrong with them. Each of the five components has identifiable symptomatology associated with it, even though not present in every case. Explain the patient's examination findings using the five components as an outline. This results in a clearer, more concise report of findings without the usual tangents and meanderings.

Using the five components as a guide avoids the X-ray view box monologue that plagues all too many reports. After all the hand waving and explanations of gas bubbles in the intestines, most patients emerge from your X-ray explanation with one major idea: bone out of place. This perception sabotages the notion of long term care because most patients can tell that you "put the bone back" on their first adjustment. They could even hear it!

Doctors using the component basis for their reports spend less time dealing with symptoms and more time focused on the patient's real problem and its correction.

4. It describes what Doctors of Chiropractic treat. In the past, the strength of chiropractic has been largely based on a strong philosophical foundation and the successful relief of pain and other symptoms. When combined with this new scientific reality, today's Doctor of Chiropractic has an exciting opportunity to change a patient's health attitude.

First, by pointing to these components, doctors can make a strong case that they don't treat "headaches" or low back pain" or other obvious spinal-related conditions. "I'm delighted you've consulted our office Mrs. Jones, however you need to know we don't treat the symptoms that you've presented here. We help locate and reduce the Vertebral Subluxation Complex, the underlying cause of a variety of health problems. Let me explain..."

Secondly, since pain or other obvious symptoms may not always be present when the Vertebral Subluxation Complex exists, it can be an excellent springboard for confronting the prevailing health attitude that the lack of symptoms means you're healthy. Relating the Vertebral Subluxation Complex to cancer or heart disease, while pointing out the bone spurs and disc narrowing that have gone undetected for years, puts needed chiropractic care in the proper framework.

5. Simplifies depositions. If you've done any personal injury work you know how the medical "experts" called on by the insurance company like to pounce on the pinched nerve model of chiropractic. And with good reason. Research suggests that 15% or less of chiropractic cases present themselves with a compressive lesion. The more common facilitative lesion has an entirely different physiology.

Even worse, when chiropractors are asked to show the "pinched nerve" on X- rays, the diagnostic tool many chiropractors hang their hats on, they can't. Of course they can't. X-rays only show the osseous component (spinal kinesiopathology—abnormal motion or position of spinal bones).

Abandoning the old "subluxation" model in favor of the Vertebral Subluxation Complex is not only more accurate, it can avoid much of the legal arena confrontation a generation of chiropractors have experienced.

6. It provides a model for the necessity of wellness care. Mitch Kapor who wrote one of the most successful programs ever, the Lotus 1-2-3 spreadsheet software, observed that "If you can genuinely present a picture that makes sense to people that unifies the seemingly separate elements of their experience; if you can give people something that they can resonate with because it's meaningful to them, they'll be immensely responsive to it." If a subluxation is a bone out of place, pinching a nerve, how come "it keeps going out?" Until you supply the explanation of long term muscle damage, soft tissue damage, and joint degeneration that accompanies aberrant spinal biomechanics, chiropractic care beyond pain relief doesn't make sense.

While Doctors of Chiropractic can take comfort in the existence of research that proves what they've known all along, substantial benefits can be reaped by developing communication strategies for sharing this information with patients.

Doctors unaware of the component basis of the Vertebral Subluxation Complex will be interested to read further.

W. H. Kirkaldy-Willis, M.A., M.D., F.R.C.S., *Managing Low Back Pain*, Churchill-Livingstone, 1988.

Abraham Towbin, M.D. Neuropathologist, Harvard Medical School,

Latent Spinal Cord and Brain Stem Injury in Newborn Infants, Develop. Med. Child Neurol., II:54-86, 1969.

Dvorak & Dovark, M.D., *Manual Medicine*, Thieme-Straton, 1984.

F. J. Kottke, M.D., G. K. Stillwell, M.D., J. F. Lehmann, M. D., Krusen's *Handbook of Physical Medicine and Rehabilitation*, W.B. Sanders Co., 1982.

J. A. Gould, III, P.T., G. J. Davies, P.T., *Orthopedic and Sports Physical Therapy*, Volume II, C. V. Mosby Co., 1985.

Alf Brieg, M.D., *Adverse Mechanical Tension of the Central Nervous System*, John Wiley & Sons, 1978.

Beighton, Grahme, Bird, M.D.'s, *Hypermobility of Joints*, Springer-Verlag, 1983.

Augustus White, III, Manohar Panjabi, *Clinical Biomechanics of the Spine,* J. B. Lippincott Co., 1978.

Karel Lewit, M.D., Sc. D., *Manipulative Therapy in Rehabilitation of the Locomotor System*, Butterworth's Publishing Co., 1985. ■

PATIENT EDUCATION
FOR THE 1990S.

Educated patients are more likely to comply with your recommendations, get well faster, remain under maintenance care, and be better equipped to tell others about chiropractic. At a time when insurance coverage is dwindling and advertising has become less effective, helping your current patients understand and vouch for their decision to seek care in your office is more important than ever. After all, if they knew what you knew, they'd do what you do. They would adopt a chiropractic lifestyle, bring their kids in for care, and tell everyone they know about chiropractic. But they don't. Even patients for whom you've worked a "miracle cure" seem unwilling to tell others.

It takes more than great results to have a great practice.

Walking into most offices these days are members of the baby boom generation. A generation raised by television. A generation that grew up with Howdy Doody, Ben Casey, Marcus Welby, and Walter Cronkite. This is a generation accustomed to getting information spoon fed by captivating visuals. We didn't read about the Kennedy assassination, we watched it on television. We didn't read about Neil Armstrong's first steps on the moon, we watched it on television. And we still don't rush home to read the newspaper. The "fireside chat" days of radio are gone. Today we turn on the tube.

Unfortunately, the communication efforts in most chiropractic offices are out of step with the new generation of chiropractic patient. It means you need to be more visual in your patient education. It almost certainly suggests the need to use video. It means modifying your report of findings. It means change!

Video-based patient education has been around since the very early 1980s. Today, you can choose from dozens of video programs. If you've tried video before and were disappointed, or you're contemplating embracing the Information Age by adding a VCR to your patient education arsenal, here are some considerations when previewing the countless patient education videos available for your office.

The video(s) must be short. Common sense suggests that you should avoid showing videos to patients in pain. Patients who are not distracted by their symptoms should be shown a video on their first visit. The purpose of this introductory video should be to orient them to a chiropractic perspective and anticipate their concerns. Moreover, it should be short. Avoid documentary length videos or presentations that are too philosophical or longer than 10 minutes. Longer than 10 minutes and your imposition may preclude their willingness to see subsequent videos. Select a first visit video that anticipates a typical patient's concerns and puts them at ease. Save the chiropractic science and philosophy for future visits.

The videos must be relevant. Patient education videos shouldn't overload the patient by numbing them with too much information. They should present relevant information as it is needed by the patient. It's inappropriate to explain the value or necessity of maintenance or wellness care on the first couple of visits. You haven't earned the right to broach this topic until you've proven you can help them with the complaint they've originally presented. Help put the common myths and misconceptions about chiropractic to rest. Deal with the doctor's education, X-rays, what an adjustment is, and their other concerns in a positive, non-defensive way.

The videos must avoid scare tactics. A previous generation could be "managed" into compliance or "scared" into compliance. Not today. The baby boom generation wants understandable information so they can make an informed decision. Recognize that ultimately patients control compliance. Their own "internal doctor" decides whether they trust you and if their condition is worth the time and money required to follow your recommendations. Present the facts clearly and without bias, honoring your patients regardless of their decisions. Take a purely informational approach and anticipate their "why?" questions. Why does it hurt? Why will it take time? Why should children seek chiropractic care? Why does it take more than one adjustment?

The videos must be highly visual. Avoid what television specialists call the "talking head" at all cost! This is the major flaw with most patient education videos, whether produced professionally with a Hollywood star, or done on a shoestring by the doctor. You might as well create an audio cassette! Putting a talking head on television is like using a highly-complex computer as a simple adding machine. It doesn't take full advantage of the compelling power of video. Patient education video should show patients things they couldn't see in any other way. We are visual animals and we get most of our information through our eyes. We remember images much longer than words. Hardly anyone remembers the words spoken by evangelist Jimmy Swagart—we remember the anguish on his tearful face.

The videos must be contemporary. Videos for patients must embrace the latest model of chiropractic and give them a complete understanding of the full nature and severity of their condition. Explaining the Vertebral Subluxation Complex is a good start. When patients understand their problem is more serious than a bone out of place (one or two visits) or a pinched nerve (discontinue care when symptoms improve), their willingness to follow through is increased. Patients are more responsive and have a greater respect for the doctor when they can visualize the seriousness of their condition. Without this understanding they can only depend on how they feel.

The videos must be part of a system. Besides making chiropractic information more visual and memorable, patient education videos should help avoid repetitious explanations. Videos should impart basic information that every patient should know, regardless of their condition. Moreover, video should be part of a multi-media effort that includes written and aural messages to allow for differing learning styles. This coordinated "systematic" approach makes patient education efforts consistent. Advertisers have long known the importance of a single, consistent message in print and broadcast media. The total impact is greater than its parts.

The videos must be supported by the staff. When patients enter a strange new environment like your office, they are extremely sensitive to the subtle, non-verbal communication of the staff. Not only should the staff see and understand every visual and every word of your video system, they must totally agree with the importance of exposing every patient to it. If staff members expect resistance when explaining to patients that "The doctor would like you to see a short video..." then they will almost certainly get it. This is the same self-fulfilling prophecy that affects patient compliance, collections, and other aspects of the doctor/patient relationship.

Video will never be a substitute or replace good old-fashioned low tech talking with patients. However, it is excellent at reducing repetitious explanations and dramatically conveying bulk amounts of basic information quickly and consistently. It can free up the doctor and staff so they can be more productive and provide better patient care. The key is to build on the information presented in your video. Reference scenes or important phrases on subsequent patient visits. Avoid the patient perception that you used the video as a momentary "babysitter." Make sure patients know the importance that you place on the video by correlating pertinent information to each patient's case.

The fact is, at the helm of the most successful practices is a doctor who is a great communicator. Regardless of adjusting technique, what school you graduated from, whether you were the oldest son or the youngest daughter, tall or thin, practice in a big city or a small town, the better your communication skills—the better your practice.

There was a time when brochures, lectures, and a monologue in front of the X-ray view box was enough. These communication technologies worked for a generation that grew up on radio and put doctors (and others with college educations) on a pedestal. Today, mere words are not the most effective way to communicate effectively with patients. Memorizing a super-duper-this-will-convince-them report of findings isn't the answer either. Better pictures are the answer. The doctor with the best pictures wins. And that most assuredly means some type of video. ■

CHIROPRACTIC DENTISTRY

It wasn't that long ago that dentists were perceived as bad teeth doctors. There was no reason or motivation to go to a dentist unless you had pain in your mouth. Perceived as just a notch above barbers, dentists were scorned, feared, and were only consulted as a last resort. It was time to see the dentist when the treatment was thought to be less painful than the inflammation caused from dental neglect.

Sounds a lot like chiropractic.

Dentistry changed. But it didn't happen overnight. Someone had the vision and the profession had the cohesiveness to implement a plan that changed the perception of the profession.

Most of us show up once or twice a year for maintenance (wellness) dentistry care. A teeth cleaning and examination that may or may not include X-rays is pretty standard operating procedure for most of us. And if someone were to warn us that "once you start seeing a dentist you have to go for the rest of your life," we'd all agree, "Of course." If we were told that there were certain preventive procedures we could do at home (up to three times a day) our compliance level, for most of us, would be quite high. Maybe not after *every* meal, but at least after *most* meals. Today, proper dental hygiene is commonly known and regularly practiced by the majority of the population.

The result? Today our population benefits from the healthiest teeth and gums of probably any time in history. The general public understands what causes tooth decay and how to prevent it. Dentists are thought of as real doctors and treated with respect. No one questions the educational achievements or competency of dentists. Paraprofessionals are trained, licensed, and work beside Doctors of Dentistry. Patients set specific appointments and, for the most part, honor them. Dentists are rarely the butt of jokes on TV situational comedies. Dentists have "come up in the world" in the last 20 or 30 years. What happened?

If chiropractic were to use the dentistry model as a cue to revamp its own image, it would first have to adopt a long term vision of the future. Advertising, *Reader's Digest* inserts, Super Bowl football star endorsements, and a lawsuit against the A.M.A. are not the solution. That's been tried. And while there's been some forward movement, it's not in the same league as the dentistry success story that's taken more than a generation to unfold. Short term solutions must be abandoned. Is the chiropractic profession ready to get behind a 10 year public relations program?

The chiropractic profession will need to have a new sense of vision and the tolerance to set aside philosophical differences. It's hard to understand the bigotry and holier-than-thou attitude held by doctors who wish to exclude, restrict, or judge the philosophy and procedures of others. It may be easier to agree on what constitutes an impacted wisdom tooth then what constitutes appropriate care for a hot low back. It may be the "art" and "philosophy" and the differences they naturally create that will ultimately preclude chiropractic from having the cohesiveness necessary to change its public perception. Certainly dentistry has its artists and philosophers too. However they were able to concentrate on what they had in common, instead of their differences. Are you big enough, self-confident enough, and trusting enough to do the same?

Let's think big. Maybe the profession could get together. If so, it will require a coordinated plan that will almost certainly have to start with children. Just like the dentistry model, you start at the beginning and work your way up. Can a profession accustomed to thinking in 90-day recovery cycles commit and follow through on a plan that may take 15 to 20 years to payoff? Can a profession that claws through the mail looking for insurance checks commit itself to helping children?

Are you prepared to launch a school education program with the same intensity that the dentists did in the elementary school I went to? After all, some other doctor may be the one to reap the rewards! Are you ready to dedicate some of your free time to explaining chiropractic to kids who respond quickly and probably aren't covered by an insurance plan? Are you equipped to explain chiropractic in terms a 10 year old can understand? Are you willing to trust an outcome that only the next generation of chiropractors will benefit from? Are you prepared to give back to your profession at the same, but different level that sent your predecessors to prison in the 1930s and '40s? Just how deep is your commitment to chiropractic?

The highest calling of any doctor is to prevent what he or she treats.

It started with free toothbrushes at school. School assemblies in which we 6th graders saw entertaining skits about the evil Sugar Monster and learned of the perils of dental neglect. Seeds were planted that took years to sprout and flourish. Are you willing to make that kind of investment in your community? Are you willing to delay the gratification? Can you assume the purity of motive to give your time and talent so the next generation of chiropractor can benefit as today's dentist is benefiting? What kind of profession will you be bequeathing to the next generation of chiropractors?

While it seems unlikely you'll go to jail for practicing chiropractic, many chiropractors today are in a different kind of prison. Probably much like the frustration that turn-of-the-century dentists experienced. Imagine what a burden it must have been to have known the value of preventive dental care and yet be sentenced to a daily grind of removing decayed teeth and being known as the deliverer of the most painful health care of last resort. To be misunderstood and unrespected creates a sense of isolation that can sabotage one's self-esteem and call into question one's purpose and chosen career.

Sound familiar?

Chiropractic needs a plan. Just who would organize and bring a plan to fruition? The national organizations? Doubtful since we can't agree on the basics. State associations and societies? Unlikely, since some states have two or three battling factions. Seminar lecturers and adjusting table entrepreneurs? Interestingly, they're about the only ones who don't ask or judge one's political persuasion. Yet, they are the ones least likely to benefit from a profession that was unified!

Until a national coalition emerges, here are some ideas you might consider in planting your own seeds for a more respected profession:

1. Become comfortable adjusting children. Become familiar with the research of Towbin and Winsor that illustrates the benefits pediatric chiropractic can have. There are several seminar programs that teach diagnostic and adjusting techniques related to newborns, infants, and children. Compare notes with doctors who already have a sizable family practice. Confront your fears.

2. Make a place in your practice for children. Before more children will show up to be patients, you may need to modify your office environment and fee structure. Get a toy box and fill it with interesting toys. Get on your hands and knees and tour your office. It looks considerably different, even foreboding at this height. Child proof your office so children are safe. Make it affordable for parents to have their children checked.

3. Design an outreach program for your community. There are a million things you can do to take chiropractic to children. Offer pre-school groups a tour of your office. Get involved with a school scoliosis screening program. Participate in the high school vocational day. Keep your motives clean! You do this because it's the right thing to do, not because you need or hope you'll get new patients.

4. Learn a new language. Ever try to explain chiropractic to a 10 year old? Practice ways of explaining what you do without using big words like subluxation, adjustment, and interference. After learning simpler ways to explain chiropractic it will probably help you communicate with adults!

Offices that work with kids seem to be having more fun. They have educated their patients and patients trust them. There's enthusiasm and vision that seems to reduce staff turnover. These are offices that seem to spawn a lot of chiropractic college students. There's a sense of purpose that prompts more referrals. There are a lot of patients who show up once or twice a month to enjoy the benefits of a chiropractic lifestyle. In short, it's a practice that has transcended into a form of chiropractic dentistry. ■

THE PARABLE OF
THE TWO TREES

Once upon a time there were two trees standing tall and proud in the midst of a beautiful meadow. The tallest tree was a perfectly proportioned fir tree. It's long needles were a *mix* of deep greens. Its bark was rough, providing easy footing for the birds, squirrels, and other forest animals it sheltered.

The other tree was a stunning maple tree with huge leaves that screamed technicolor sunsets in the fall. Its bark was smooth and its branches reached *straight* out in fingers that poked at the sky. The strong trunk and branches bent easily in the wind as its leaves fluttered like feathers.

One summer day as both trees stood surveying the green carpeted meadow below they struck up a conversation. To have two trees talking, well, that was pretty unusual. But in this case their conversation was even more incredible because of the almost 100 years of silence that they had stood side by side without speaking.

"Kind of a rough winter this time," observed the fir tree speaking first.

"I hadn't noticed," said the maple, "it's always difficult when one loses all of one's leaves. I don't have the insurance of a thick green coat of needles like you do."

"Yeah, I help a lot of forest animals because of the protection my branches offer," said the fir tree proudly. "Why I had two owls and several squirrels this year."

"That's nice, but the maple syrup I provided was on the breakfast tables of several human families," proclaimed the maple, straightening up and standing a bit more erectly.

"There you go again with your 'I'm-better-than-you' attitude!" shouted the fir. "How can a tree that loses it leaves and stands there naked each winter, exposed to the elements, be considered superior to a noble fir tree?"

After this outburst both trees fell silent, thinking about the conversation and why each thought the other was inferior. While each was in deep thought the weather changed. A looming thundercloud filled the summer sky and burst above them releasing big drops of water, which quickly turned to hail.

When the sky stopped falling both trees stood in a quarry of cold white gravel. The melting ice dropped from the boughs of the fir tree. Next to the fir tree, with its leaves shredded below it like taco lettuce in sour cream, stood the nude maple.

Again, the fir was the first to break the silence.

"That was quite a storm."

"I've experienced worse," sniffed the maple.

"What are you going to do?" asked the fir who was now feeling a little guilty for having better weathered the storm.

"The same thing I always do," snapped the maple with greater resolve. I've already started growing new leaves."

"Why don't you just grow needles like I do?" volunteered the fir trying to help.

"Are you kidding? I don't believe in needles. Needles are for trees that take the easy way out. Oh, I could grow needles if I wanted to, but I think it distracts from the real purpose of being a tree," proclaimed the maple bluntly.

"What do you mean?" asked the fir tree trying to understand. "Everyone expects needles. If I didn't have needles I couldn't help the birds and all the animals that seek shelter from me. Without my needles I'd disappoint them."

"That's only because you've never experienced what it feels like to see your seeds helicopter to the far corners of the meadow," glowed the maple.

The fir paused to collect his thoughts.

"But just look at you!" laughed the fir. "What good are you now without your leaves?"

"Ah, but I trust in my potential to grow more leaves," smiled the maple with assurance.

The fir tree thought about that for a moment. He'd never lost all his needles before and really wasn't convinced they'd grow back if he somehow lost them. In fact, he'd never given much thought to his needles or why someone would prefer the more difficult decision to grow leaves.

The fir tree's musings were interrupted by a large owl that landed in one of his upper branches.

"We all couldn't help but notice the two of you arguing," said the owl speaking to no one in particular, but loud enough for both trees to hear. "What's the problem?"

"I was just explaining the virtues of leaves and the inborn potential to grow new ones," answered the maple.

"And I was just explaining why it's easier to grow needles," said the fir.

"Why not have both leaves and needles," suggested the owl trying to make peace.

"That's a good idea," said the fir tree brightening at the obvious solution.

"Impossible!" cried the maple. "You'd lose all sense of 'tree-ness' if you did that."

Unperturbed the owl ventured into even deeper water. "Why not outlaw one or the other? Pass a law or make it especially difficult for the weaker or less correct tree to survive."

There. It was out in the open. Both trees went deep into thought after the owl had verbalized the unmentionable. It was this central issue of "rightness" that had started the stand off so many years earlier. Each could see the other's contribution to the ecological balance of the meadow, but neither was willing to confront the either/or position advanced by the owl. They rather liked the competition and the passion generated by their differences. They realized that too much of their outlook on life as a tree was defined by the desire to show off their own "purity" or "open-mindedness." Regardless of who became king of the forest, they both sensed that something would be missing without the diversity represented by the other.

By now the sun had set and the meadow was dark and quiet except for a few birds settling down to rest for the night. Not even the moon shined through the remaining overcast skies above.

"Are you asleep yet?" whispered the fir tree.

"No, are you?" answered the maple.

"I've been thinking," volunteered the fir, "about what the owl said earlier. I think you're a great tree. I guess I've always been kind of envious. You always seem to have the passion and the commitment I wish I had."

After a short pause the maple responded, "Thanks. I guess I've always been jealous of your success in attracting and helping all the forest animals. You always seem so easy going and don't see things as black or white."

"I wish I could experience the simplicity and focus of having leaves," confessed the fir.

"I wonder what it's like to have a green coat all year long," said the maple rather dreamily.

The two trees started talking. All through the dark night they talked and talked. Though they couldn't see each other, they gained strength from their new understanding of each other. They talked of their common enemies, forest fires, early freezes, hungry wintertime deer, and invading insects. By morning the conversation got quite lively as they shared their fears, their dreams of the future, and the collected wisdom of being a tree for almost a hundred years. The more they talked the more they realized how much they had in common. They discovered how superficial leaves and needles really are.

* * *

The struggle over win/lose, either/or, right/wrong, and we/them has distracted too many for too long. Bigotry in any form, divides and prepares the soil for conquest. Those who cannot tolerate others are revealing a mistrust of their own beliefs. That fragile commodity called "intelligence" that chiropractors deal with is measured by its ability to adapt. Adapting is not to be confused with compromise. To adapt, one moves forward in spite of the obstacle. Adapting honors the barrier or challenge and continues forward with a new homeostatic balance. Adaptation is fundamentally win/win.

To compromise one gives up or sells out to create a muddy gray area which pleases no one. A compromise tends to weaken the strong in the hopes of bolstering the weak. It never works. A compromise is almost always lose/lose.

Maybe if the conversation alfresco had taken place years earlier the bulldozers that leveled both trees in the meadow for a new regional medical center could have been avoided. Maybe the subject of trees would have been more widely taught in public schools. Maybe the trees wouldn't be such easy targets for media pundits. Maybe trees would garner the respect they deserve. Maybe. ■

ADDITIONAL RESOURCES

Every author receives inspiration from others and being a voracious reader myself, perhaps you would like to review some of the influences that helped create this book. Here is a partial list of the most recent books that contributed to this volume:

Positively Outrageous Service, by T. Scott Gross. Recognizing that extraordinary service is the key to building positive word of mouth, Mr. Gross shows you ways some different types of businesses do it. A "business book" that's practical and very readable.

At the Leading Edge, by Michael Toms. This is a thoughtful book of 14 essays, that tackles some of today's most interesting ethical, scientific, and social issues. These are transcripts of some great interviews from Michael Tom's National Public Radio program that make easy reading.

Revolution From Within, by Gloria Steinem. Abandon all the dogma about Gloria Steinem from her militant feminist past! This is a delightful book about self-esteem. Since your practice never outgrows your self-esteem, I'll be recommending this book for years to come!

Live and Learn and Pass it On, by H. Jackson Brown, Jr. A contemporary *Book of Proverbs*. People ages five to 95 were asked what they had "learned" over their lives. It's upbeat tone is perfect for the reception room. (Rutledge Hill Press, 513 Third Ave South, Nashville, TN 37210)

The Customer Comes Second, by Hal Rosenbluth. The title caught my eye because we're accustomed to thinking the customer/patient comes first. Using the backdrop of the largest travel agency in the world, Mr. Rosenbluth demonstrates why your staff comes first because your staff treats your customer the same way you treat your staff!

Inner Excellence, Spiritual Principles of a Life-Driving Business by Carol Orsborn. A powerful book with insights into why we are tempted to work harder instead of smarter. Learn ways of extricating yourself from perfectionism and develop a better balance between work and play. Reclaim your life!

You've Got To Be Believed To Be Heard by Bert Decker. This is an excellent communication book that will give you an exciting understanding of better ways to reach patients. Finally explains why great communicators have better compliance, more fun, and bigger practices.

230

Sur/Petition, Going Beyond Competition by Edward DeBono. All of DeBono's books are excellent sources for creative thinking models. In this one he details methods for transcending competitive forces and creating monopolies of value that create long term customer relationships.

Information Anxiety by Richard Wurman. A beautifully crafted book that explains why patients don't respond to most reports of findings. It offers constructive ideas for the better presentation of information. Just reading the annotations along the edges of the pages is inspirational!

Follow The Yellow Brick Road by Richard Wurman. This follow-up book focuses entirely on the process of giving, taking, and using directions. He covers the five basic components of effective instructions. Prepare to rework your report of findings after browsing through this one.

The Art of Self-Renewal by Dr. Barbara Mackoff. Are you tempted to take the most frustrating and disrespectful patients home with you? Do you feel you're working harder but getting further behind? Here are some suggestions for balancing the pressures of work and family and improving both in the process.

The Popcorn Report by Faith Popcorn. Ms. Popcorn is the Alvin Toffler and John Naisbitt of the 1990s. Her consulting firm specializes in advising *Fortune* 500 corporations on significant consumer trends that may affect their business, products, and services.

Personal Styles & Effective Performance by David Merrill and Roger Reid. If you're an Analytical or Amiable personality, you'll especially enjoy this insightful book that explains many of the communication difficulties these two quadrants experience and what to do about it. If you're an Expressive like about 75% of the chiropractic profession, you'll understand why banker-types drive you crazy!

Unlimited Power by Anthony Robbins. This is the book that launched his audio cassette programs and continuous TV infomercials. Besides putting NLP concepts in laymen's terms, read this classic for a lot of practical recipes for advancing personal change.

Compassion International Child Sponsorship. I've traveled extensively overseas for this Christian child sponsorship program and I'm impressed with their work, their financial accountability, and low overhead. To help a child escape the cycle of poverty contact them at Compassion International, P.O. Box 7000, Colorado Springs, CO 80933, or call (719) 594-9900.

William Esteb provides a variety of seminars, consulting services, and patient education tools to enhance practice growth through Back Talk Systems, Inc. Call or write for a catalog of practice aids that reflect his patient-centered philosophy and to receive *The Patient's Point of View* newsletter. Mr. Esteb is available for in office consultations and speaking engagements and can be contacted at Back Talk Systems, Inc. for more information.

Back Talk Systems, Inc.
2845 Ore Mill Drive, Suite 4
Colorado Springs, CO 80904-3161
(800) 937-3113